T0259353

Cardiovascular Rheumatic Diseases

Editor

RICHARD D. BRASINGTON Jr

RHEUMATIC DISEASE CLINICS OF NORTH AMERICA

www.rheumatic.theclinics.com

Consulting Editor
MICHAEL H. WEISMAN

February 2014 • Volume 40 • Number 1

ELSEVIER

1600 John F. Kennedy Boulevard • Suite 1800 • Philadelphia, Pennsylvania, 19103-2899
http://www.theclinics.com

RHEUMATIC DISEASE CLINICS OF NORTH AMERICA Volume 40, Number 1
February 2014 ISSN 0889-857X, ISBN 13: 978-0-323-29700-4

Editor: Jennifer Flynn-Briggs
Developmental Editor: Susan Showalter

Rheumatic Disease Clinics of North America (ISSN 0889-857X) is published quarterly by Elsevier Inc., 360 Park Avenue South, New York, NY 10010-1710. Months of issue are February, May, August, and November. Business and editorial offices: 1600 John F. Kennedy Boulevard, Suite 1800, Philadelphia, PA 19103-2899. Periodicals postage paid at New York, NY and additional mailing offices. Subscription prices are USD 335.00 per year for US individuals, USD 579.00 per year for US institutions, USD 165.00 per year for US students and residents, USD 395.00 per year for Canadian individuals, USD 722.00 per year for Canadian institutions, USD 465.00 per year for international individuals, USD 722.00 per year for international institutions, and USD 230.00 per year for Canadian and foreign students/residents. To receive student/resident rate, orders must be accompanied by name of affiliated institution, date of term, and the *signature* of program/residency coordinator on institution letterhead. Orders will be billed at individual rate until proof of status received. Foreign air speed delivery is included in all *Clinics* subscription prices. All prices are subject to change without notice. **POSTMASTER:** Send address changes to *Rheumatic Disease Clinics of North America,* Elsevier Health Sciences Division, Subscription Customer Service, 3251 Riverport Lane, Maryland Heights, MO 63043. **Customer Service: 1-800-654-2452 (US and Canada). From outside of the US and Canada: 314-447-8871. Fax: 314-447-8029. For print support,** e-mail: **JournalsCustomerService-usa@elsevier.com. For online support, e-mail: JournalsOnline Support-usa@elsevier.com.**

Reprints. For copies of 100 or more of articles in this publication, please contact the Commercial Reprints Department, Elsevier Inc., 360 Park Avenue South, New York, New York, 10010-1710; Tel.: +1-212-633-3874, Fax: +1-212-633-3820, and E-mail: reprints@elsevier.com.

Rheumatic Disease Clinics of North America is covered in MEDLINE/PubMed (Index Medicus), Current Contents/Clinical Medicine, Science Citation Index, ISI/BIOMED, and EMBASE/Excerpta Medica.

Printed and bound by CPI Group (UK) Ltd, Croydon, CR0 4YY

Transferred to digital print 2013

Contributors

CONSULTING EDITOR

MICHAEL H. WEISMAN, MD
Division of Rheumatology, Cedars-Sinai Medical Center, Los Angeles, California

EDITOR

RICHARD D. BRASINGTON Jr, MD
Professor, Division of Rheumatology, Department of Medicine, Washington University School of Medicine in St Louis, St Louis, Missouri

AUTHORS

SAMAN AHMED, MD
MICU Hospitalist, Medical Intensive Care Unit, Department of Medicine, Penn Presbyterian Medical Center, University of Pennsylvania Health System, Philadelphia, Pennsylvania

KEVIN BASZIS, MD
Division of Rheumatology, Department of Pediatrics, Washington University School of Medicine, St Louis, Missouri

VIDULA BHOLE, MD
Palo Alto, California

RICHARD D. BRASINGTON Jr, MD
Professor, Division of Rheumatology, Department of Medicine, Washington University School of Medicine in St Louis, St Louis, Missouri

CHRISTINA CHARLES-SCHOEMAN, MD, MS
Division of Rheumatology, Department of Medicine, University of California Los Angeles, Los Angeles, California

LAMPROS FOTIS, MD, PhD
Division of Rheumatology, Department of Pediatrics, Washington University School of Medicine, St Louis, Missouri

HOWARD VAN GELDER, MD
Rheumatology Fellow, Division of Rheumatology, Department of Internal Medicine, Olive View-UCLA Medical Center, Los Angeles, California

MARÍA GONZÁLEZ-MAYDA, MD
Instructor, Division of Rheumatology, Department of Medicine, Washington University School of Medicine, St Louis, Missouri

ALFRED H.J. KIM, MD, PhD
Instructor, Division of Rheumatology, Department of Medicine, Washington University School of Medicine, St Louis, Missouri

MALEEWAN KITCHAROENSAKKUL, MD
Division of Rheumatology, Allergy and Immunology, Department of Pediatrics,
Washington University School of Medicine, St Louis, Missouri

ESWAR KRISHNAN, MD, M.Phil
ARAMIS Program, Department of Medicine, Stanford University, Palo Alto, California

ELI MILOSLAVSKY, MD
Rheumatology Unit, Division of Rheumatology, Allergy, and Immunology, Department of
Medicine, Massachusetts General Hospital, Boston, Massachusetts

JONATHAN J. MINER, MD, PhD
Fellow, Division of Rheumatology, Department of Medicine, Washington University
School of Medicine, St Louis, Missouri

HAROLD I. PALEVSKY, MD
Professor of Medicine, Chief, Pulmonary, Allergy and Critical Care Medicine, Director,
Pulmonary Vascular Disease Program, Penn Presbyterian Medical Center, Perelman
School of Medicine, University of Pennsylvania, Philadelphia, Pennsylvania

JOHN L. PARKS, MD
Fellow, Division of Cardiology, Medical University of South Carolina, Charleston,
South Carolina

LAURA P. PARKS, MD
Fellow, Division of Rheumatology and Immunology, Medical University of South Carolina,
Charleston, South Carolina

DEEPALI SEN, MBBS
Assistant Professor, Division of Rheumatology, Department of Medicine, Washington
University School of Medicine, St Louis, Missouri

RICHARD M. SILVER, MD
Distinguished University Professor, Division of Rheumatology and Immunology, Medical
University of South Carolina, Charleston, South Carolina

MARIAN H. TAYLOR, MD
Assistant Professor of Medicine, Division of Cardiology, Medical University of South
Carolina, Charleston, South Carolina

SEBASTIAN UNIZONY, MD
Rheumatology Unit, Division of Rheumatology, Allergy, and Immunology, Department of
Medicine, Massachusetts General Hospital, Boston, Massachusetts

TIPHANIE VOGEL, MD, PhD
Division of Rheumatology, Departments of Pediatrics and Medicine, Washington
University School of Medicine, St Louis, Missouri

Contents

defects, valvular disease, and coronary artery disease. In addition to cardiac disease in adults with SLE, the children of women with SLE can develop neonatal lupus by passive transfer of autoantibodies across the placenta. This article describes the cardiac manifestations of SLE and highlights some key unanswered questions about the disease and its pathogenesis.

Recent advances in Kawasaki disease have included attempts to define genes involved in its pathogenesis. There have been recent advances in the studies of rheumatic carditis, leading to a better understanding of the mechanism of the disease. Histologic evaluation of patients with neonatal lupus erythematosus has revealed fibrosis with collagen deposition and calcification of the atrioventricular node. Therapy for cardiac involvement in systemic juvenile idiopathic arthritis should involve treatment of the underlying disease and systemic inflammatory state, and typically includes nonsteroidal antiinflammatory drugs, corticosteroids, disease-modifying drugs, and biologic therapies targeting tumor necrosis factor-alpha, interleukin-1, and interleukin-6.

Heart disease, either clinically apparent or silent, is a frequent complication of systemic sclerosis (SSc, scleroderma) and may affect both patients with diffuse cutaneous and limited cutaneous SSc. The availability of more sensitive modalities has led to an increased awareness of scleroderma heart disease, which often involves the pericardium, myocardium, and cardiac conduction system. This awareness of cardiac involvement requires attention and interventions led by internists, cardiologists, and rheumatologists. Although no specific therapy exists for scleroderma heart disease, early recognition of the presence and type of scleroderma heart disease may lead to more effective management of patients with scleroderma.

Associated pulmonary arterial hypertension related to connective tissue disorders carries significant morbidity and a high mortality. The purpose of this review article is to present an updated account of the pathogenesis, epidemiology, clinical signs and symptoms, diagnostic modalities, treatment regimens, and prognosis of this disorder.

The association between gout and cardiovascular diseases has been noted for centuries but was not subjected to rigorous epidemiologic studies until recently. The published literature is almost unanimous in the strength and consistency of this association. However, the impact of gout over and above that conferred by hyperuricemia and other risk factors of cardiovascular disease has not been well studied. Future studies are expected to shed light on the pathophysiologic basis of this association.

RHEUMATIC DISEASE CLINICS OF NORTH AMERICA

Foreword

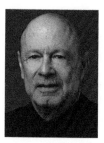

Michael H. Weisman, MD
Consulting Editor

A volume to address the concept of heart disease as a "comorbidity" related to our well-known rheumatic phenotypes is long overdue. There is no better person to put this together than Rick Brasington, a rheumatologist of great stature in the field possessing extensive experience in so many different rheumatic diseases as well as a superb clinical educator. These articles touch on cardiac involvement in a variety of our diseases with discussions about clinical presentations and mechanistic aspects. With our increasing ability to control many of the clinical features of our diseases with potent targeted therapies, this issue becomes more important. There may be choices among very powerful interventions, given early, that may impact the cardiac risks associated with these conditions. So, this volume is timely, important, and hopefully useful for patient decision-making, and we are grateful to Rick and his collaborators for putting it together.

Michael H. Weisman, MD
Division of Rheumatology
Cedars-Sinai Medical Center
8700 Beverly Boulevard
Los Angeles, CA 90024, USA

E-mail address:
michael.weisman@cshs.org

Rheum Dis Clin N Am 40 (2014) ix
http://dx.doi.org/10.1016/j.rdc.2013.10.010
0889-857X/14/$ – see front matter © 2014 Published by Elsevier Inc.

Preface

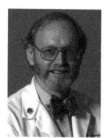

Richard D. Brasington Jr, MD
Editor

When I was in medical school, I remember arguing with a classmate about whether the brain or the heart should be considered the more important organ. My classmate declared, "The Heart is just a pump to supply the Brain with blood, so the Brain is more important." I countered that without the Heart, the Brain was dead, so I felt that I had won the argument.

Our understanding of The Heart in the Rheumatic Diseases has become much more sophisticated since my fellowship during the 1980s. Although we were then beginning to realize that the life expectancy of severe rheumatoid arthritis (RA) was similar to that of three-vessel coronary artery disease, we did not yet understand that the RA itself was a significant risk factor for coronary disease. Furthermore, during the last decade, we learned that rather than protecting against coronary disease, nonsteroidal drugs may have an adverse effect on coronary disease.

In this volume, we have gathered experts in their respective fields to review the most recent literature to help us more fully understand how the heart can be involved in the major rheumatologic disorders. Since the heart is itself a muscle, we begin with the inflammatory myopathies, in which Van Gelder and Charles-Schoeman focuses on myocarditis and cardiomyopathies. Unizony and Miloslavsky follow with a thorough inventory of cardiac involvement in the systemic vasculitides.

Sen and Gonzalez-Mayda bring us up to date on our current understanding of the heart in RA: not only coronary disease, but pericarditis, valvular heart disease, and the myocardial effects of medications used to treat RA. Baszis and colleagues address pediatric rheumatic diseases, covering juvenile arthritis and dermatomyositis, acute rheumatic fever, and Kawasaki disease.

The multiple cardiac manifestations of lupus are covered by Miner and Kim, who concentrate on neonatal lupus, pericarditis, myocarditis, and the very complex issue of premature coronary artery disease in lupus patients. The scleroderma section by Parks and colleagues is followed by a thorough treatment of pulmonary artery hypertension by Ahmed and Palevsky, emphasizing the fact that pulmonary hypertension is the leading cause of death in scleroderma. These articles discuss the most current methods for detecting and following pulmonary hypertension, a rapidly evolving field.

Rheum Dis Clin N Am 40 (2014) xi–xii
http://dx.doi.org/10.1016/j.rdc.2013.10.009
0889-857X/14/$ – see front matter © 2014 Published by Elsevier Inc.

rheumatic.theclinics.com

We conclude with gout, a condition for which rheumatologists are much more focused on the joints than the myocardium. Krishnan reminds us that there is much more to gout than just arthritis.

Our goal has been to gather together in one volume the state of the art of what is known about the heart in the rheumatic diseases in 2014. We hope that this will be of value to students at all levels, as well as practitioners of rheumatology.

Richard D. Brasington Jr, MD
Division of Rheumatology
Washington University in St Louis
156 Gray Avenue
St Louis, MO 63119-2914, USA

E-mail address:
richard.brasington@sbcglobal.net

The Heart in Inflammatory Myopathies

Howard Van Gelder, MD[a],
Christina Charles-Schoeman, MD, MS[b],*

KEYWORDS

- Idiopathic inflammatory myopathies • Cardiovascular disease • Dermatomyositis
- Polymyositis • Inclusion body myositis

KEY POINTS

- Systemic autoimmune diseases are becoming increasingly linked to accelerated risks of cardiovascular disease and events, and the idiopathic inflammatory myopathies (IIM) are not an exception to this growing pattern.
- Traditional risk factors for coronary artery disease, such as hypertension and hyperlipidemia, are associated with cardiovascular disease and events in patients with IIM.
- IIM patients with cardiac involvement are at increased risk for overall mortality when compared with IIM patients without cardiac involvement.
- The effects of immunosuppression on cardiac disease and cardiovascular events in IIM patients requires further investigation in carefully controlled studies.
- It is imperative that physicians treating IIM patients perform a routine cardiovascular risk assessment at the onset of diagnosis.

INTRODUCTION

Inflammatory muscle diseases are a diverse set of systemic autoimmune rheumatic disorders that are defined by chronic muscle weakness, muscle fatigue, and mononuclear cell infiltration into skeletal muscle. Idiopathic inflammatory myopathies (IIMs) primarily affect the trunk and proximal limb muscles with or without skin involvement.[1] There are various subtypes, including polymyositis (PM), dermatomyositis (DM), juvenile myositis, amyopathic myositis, and inclusion body myositis (IBM). The Bohan and Peter criteria have been widely used in diagnosing PM/DM (**Box 1**), however updated classification criteria for these disorders which include IBM are currently in development.[2] The reported overall incidence of IIMs is approximately 10 cases per million the United States. Diagnosis of IIMs is usually based on a combination of clinical signs

[a] Division of Rheumatology, Department of Internal Medicine, Olive View-UCLA Medical Center, Los Angeles, CA, USA; [b] Division of Rheumatology, Department of Medicine, University of California Los Angeles, 1000 Veteran Avenue, Room 32-59, Los Angeles, CA 90095, USA
* Corresponding author.
E-mail address: CCharles@mednet.ucla.edu

Rheum Dis Clin N Am 40 (2014) 1–10
http://dx.doi.org/10.1016/j.rdc.2013.10.002
0889-857X/14/$ – see front matter

Box 1
Modified Bohan and Peter criteria for the diagnosis of PM and DM

Individual criteria

1. Symmetric proximal muscle weakness

2. Muscle biopsy evidence of myositis

3. Increase in serum skeletal muscle enzymes

4. Characteristic electromyographic pattern

5. Typical rash of dermatomyositis

Diagnostic criteria

Polymyositis

　Definite: all of 1–4, Probable: any 3 of 1–4, Possible: any 2 of 1–4

Dermatomyositis

　Definite: 5 plus any 3 of 1–4, Probable: 5 plus any 2 of 1–4, Possible: 5 plus any of 1–4

Data from Oddis CV, Ascherman DP. Clinical features, classification, and epidemiology of inflammatory muscle disease. In: Hochberg M, Silman A, Smolen J, et al, editors. Rheumatology. 5th edition. New York: Elsevier; 2011.

---

and symptoms along with key laboratory and diagnostic testing. Among the important blood tests include measurements of enzyme levels expressed from damaged muscle and autoantibodies, including myositis-specific antibodies such as anti-synthetase antibodies (anti-Jo1 and others), anti-SRP, Anti-Mi2, anti-MDA5, anti-MJ, and anti-TIF1-gamma.[3] Diagnostic studies include abnormal electromyographic measurements of affected muscle, magnetic resonance imaging suggesting muscle edema, and muscle biopsy showing the characteristic abnormalities. Medical treatments generally (excluding IBM) consist of immune suppression in the form of corticosteroids followed by a variety of disease-modifying antirheumatic drugs depending on the organ systems involved.[4]

The IIMs can be complicated by many disorders of the internal organs (**Box 2**). Arthritis, gastrointestinal tract (dysphagia), skin (primarily in DM), and lung (interstitial lung disease) are among the many well-known organ systems involved with IIM. Cardiovascular disease is a risk factor for death among patients with PM and DM even though clinically evident heart involvement is rarely reported. However, many subclinical manifestations of heart disease have been reported, suggesting that clinical disease may in fact be underreported.[5] The literature evaluating the subject of cardiac involvement in IIM has not been extensive, although interest has recently increased in this area as better diagnostic tools become available and a focus on improving treatment outcomes continues. Herein, we present a brief review focused on the most recent developments in cardiovascular disease and IIM.

METHODS

Articles were searched on pubmed.gov for the keywords of "Myositis" or "IIM" or "Myopathy" with the boolean operator AND followed by "Cardiovascular Disease" or "Cardiac" or "Cardiomyopathy" and appropriate articles were chosen. Only articles in English published after 2005 were chosen for inclusion if they were deemed

---

Box 2
Organ Involvement in IIM

Muscle

- Atrophy, weakness, dysfunction

Skeletal

- Joint contracture, osteoporosis with fracture, avascular necrosis, arthropathy

Cutaneous

- Calcinosis, alopecia, scarring, pokiloderma, lipodystrophy

Gastrointestinal

- Dysphagia, dysmotility, infarction

Pulmonary

- Dysphonia, impaired lung function, pulmonary fibrosis, hypertension

Cardiovascular

- Hypertension, ventricular dysfunction, angina, myocardial infarction

Peripheral vascular disease

- Tissue pulp loss, digit loss, thrombosis, claudication

Endocrine

- Growth failure, delay in secondary sexual characteristics, hirsutism, irregular menses, amenorrhea, diabetes, infertility, sexual dysfunction

Ocular severity

- Cataract, vision loss

Infection

- Chronic infection, multiple infections

Data from National Institute of Environmental Health Sciences. IMACS Myositis Damage Index 2001. Available at: http://www.niehs.nih.gov/research/resources/assets/docs/myositis_damage_index_pdf_format.pdf. Accessed September 30, 2013.

---

to be appropriate for the current review as determined by the authors. In addition, Web searches for online textbooks in rheumatology and IIM were included besides the initial PubMed search and the same inclusion criterion was applied. Further articles were then located based on references found in the initial article or text review.

RESULTS
Cardiomyopathies: Myocarditis

Cardiomyopathies can be defined as myocardial disorders in which the heart muscle is structurally and functionally abnormal in the absence of coronary artery disease (CAD), hypertension, valvular heart disease, and congenital heart disease.[6] Cardiac magnetic resonance imaging (CMR) provides 3-dimensional data on cardiac anatomy, function, tissue characterization, coronary and microvascular perfusion, and valvular disease without ionizing radiation. Several case reports and case series have demonstrated a link between myocarditis identified by MRI and inflammatory myopathies.

In one report by Mavrogeni and colleagues,[7] 7 patients with PM and 9 patients with DM without apparent clinical symptoms, clinical risk factors, or laboratory studies of cardiac involvement were evaluated by CMR. Fourteen of the patients were in clinical remission at the time of the study. The results revealed the presence of late gadolinium enhancement in 9 of 16 patients in epicardial/intramyocardial portions of the heart. Five percent of the myocardial mass was typically involved. No direct cardiac biopsies were performed to confirm the results.

Another report found asymptomatic signs of myocarditis in the posterior and inferior walls via CMR in an adolescent with juvenile overlap-myositis treated with steroids and methotrexate.[8]

A recent study from Greece evaluated 20 newly diagnosed patients with IIM (10 DM/ 10 PM) with a median disease duration of 20 days and no known coronary artery disease (CAD). The study population was found to have evidence of myocarditis in 15 of 20 patients using CMR.[9] Reevaluation 3 months later in 12 of 15 patients following steroid therapy still showed 10 of 12 positive for myocarditis despite the disease being considered in remission.

Cardiomyopathies: Structural/Electrophysiologic Abnormalities

Data regarding structural and electrophysiologic abnormalities in patients with IIM are also emerging. A case series from Sénéchal and colleagues[10] describes a patient with longstanding DM from 1989 to 2003 found to have new onset left bundle branch block and severe systolic dysfunction despite his DM being under good clinical control, with no "clinical intercurrent flares," for nearly 14 years. The authors did note that he had abnormal CPK assessments during the course of his DM, varying between 245 U/L and 300 U/L (normal value 195 U/L or less). Cardiac biopsy demonstrated moderate myocardial fibrosis. The same authors described a case of PM in a woman with normal ejection fraction (EF) of 70% at the time of diagnosis who responded clinically to prednisone and methotrexate including normalization of her initially abnormal CPK. She presented 2 years later with palpitations and premature ventricular complexes on Holter and then went into cardiac arrest. She survived, and repeat EF was 35% with cardiac biopsy showing interstitial fibrosis.

Cardiac dysfunction has also been reported in juvenile dermatomyositis (JDM). A study by Schwartz and colleagues[11] in 2010 evaluated 59 patients with JDM compared to 59 age and sex-matched controls. Abnormalities in electrocardiography (ECG) and echocardiography were examined. Patients with JDM were all under age 18 at diagnosis, had the disease for more than 24 months, and underwent clinical examination in addition to other laboratory testing. ECG was "pathologic" in 17% of patients versus 7% of controls, with 2 study patients showing signs of left ventricular hypertrophy (LVH) by ECG criteria. Diastolic dysfunction as measured by the early diastolic transmitral flow/early diastolic tissue velocity ratio, E/E', was found in 22% of study patients versus 0% of controls at a median of 16.8 years after diagnosis. The higher the disease activity score at 1 year, the worse the diastolic dysfunction measured by the E/E'.

A series of 51 patients with sporadic IBM were evaluated in a study from the Netherlands that revealed impaired systolic function in 4 (8%) and LVH in 14 (27%) of patients. These values were not different compared to age-matched population controls,[12] leading the authors to conclude that no routine comprehensive cardiac evaluation was needed in IBM patients without cardiac symptoms. In the same study there were elevated levels of CK-MB and cardiac troponin T enzymes in IBM patients, however, those elevations did not correlate with cardiac involvement and were felt to originate from skeletal muscle tissue. Only one IBM patient with known severe cardiomyopathy had an elevated troponin I enzyme.

A case report presented a 73-year-old man with IBM without known CAD risk factors with new onset New York Heart Association class II heart failure.[13] His echocardiogram showed a decreased ejection fraction (EF) at 37%, an enlarged left ventricle, and diffuse hypokinesia. He had a negative angiogram and no other identifiable cause to explain his symptoms. Cardiac MRI confirmed left ventricle enlargement but no necrosis fibrosis, or other alterations in myocardial perfusion and architecture.

CAD and Cerebral Vascular Disease

Increased morbidity and mortality due to coronary heart disease (CHD) is well established in other rheumatic conditions such as systemic lupus erythematosus and rheumatoid arthritis. Initial work suggests a similar trend in patients with DM and PM.[14]

Linos and colleagues[15] evaluated the frequency and mortality rates of atherosclerotic cardiovascular disease (CVD) in DM patients using data from the US Nationwide Inpatient Sample (INS) from 1993 to 2007. In 50,322 hospitalizations of DM patients 20% were associated with concurrent atherosclerotic cardiovascular diagnosis or procedure. Patients with DM and atherosclerotic CVD were almost twice as likely to die in hospital as compared to age and gender matched non-DM controls with similar CVD. In addition, DM patients with CVD were twice as likely to die compared to DM patients without CVD. Congestive heart failure and CAD were the second and third most frequent diagnoses associated with DM hospitalizations following pneumonia.

Risk for coronary heart disease–related hospitalizations within a year after hospitalization for many different autoimmune disorders (including PM/DM) was evaluated in a study in Sweden published in 2012. In this study, patients hospitalized for PM/DM from 1964 to 2008 were found to have a standardized risk of hospitalization for CAD of 3.81 versus the normal population in the year after their hospitalization for DM/PM. The risk decreased over the next 10 years but remained elevated.[16] The study was limited to patients who were hospitalized for DM/PM and thus may reflect a population that is more acutely active/ill than the entire DM/PM population.

A similar study of all individuals in Sweden hospitalized with an autoimmune disease (including PM/DM) without prior cerebral vascular accident (CVA) between 1987 and 2008 were followed until their first hospitalization for ischemic or hemorrhagic CVA and compared to the population at large. The number of PM/DM admissions was greater than 400, with a standardized risk of hospitalization of CVA of all types at 1.85.[17]

Finally, Tisseverasinghe and colleagues[18] studied a cohort of DM and PM patients from Canadian administrative databases and evaluated new cases of ischemic heart disease, cerebrovascular accidents (CVA), and peripheral artery disease from billing and hospitalization data. Incident arterial events occurred in 80 patients, including 34 myocardial infarctions (13.8/1,000 person-years) and 13 CVAs (5.1/1,000 person years), which were higher than rates from the general Canadian population.

Cardiovascular Risk Factors

Higher rates of traditional cardiovascular risk factors such as diabetes and hypertension have been reported in IIM patients compared to the general population. A study of patients in an inflammatory myopathy database in Australia evaluated 43 patients with DM, 184 with PM, and 117 with IBM from 1980 to 2009 for CAD risk factors.[19] Rates of hypertension, diabetes, and other coronary risk factors were obtained through questionnaires filled out over several years of follow-up. The study did not account for onset of the risk factors before, during, or after diagnosis and treatments. Sixty-two percent of the patients had hypertension, 29% had diabetes, and 49% smoked compared to 9.4%, 4%, and 20% of controls, respectively. Hyperlipidemia of 13% was similar to controls, but in subgroup analysis was higher in IBM patients compared to DM/PM, felt related in part to the older age of the IBM population. Where data of pre-/post-diagnosis were available, the study showed a higher rate for hypertension occurring before diagnosis in IIM patients. Comparing IIM subgroups, hypertension and diabetes occurred more frequently following the diagnosis of myositis in DM patients compared to PM or IBM patients. Twenty-six percent had ischemic heart disease overall in the study.

Hypertension was also increased in a study of JDM patients in Norway. None of the 59 matched controls had hypertension compared to none of the controls.[11] In the previously mentioned Canadian study by Tisseverasinghe and colleagues, patients experiencing arterial events had higher rates of traditional risk factors, such as hypertension and hyperlipidemia. Use of non-steroid immunomodulators (methotrexate, azathioprine, antimalarial agents, and cyclophosphamide) was inversely associated with CV events.[18]

A pilot study from Chicago studied 8 adults with history of JDM (median disease duration of 29 years) who were compared to 8 healthy age-matched controls and evaluated for carotid intima media thickness and brachial arterial reactivity to assess cardiovascular risk.[20] The authors found that JDM patients had increased intima media thickness and impairment of endothelial cell function based on brachial arterial reactivity versus controls. The JDM patients also had higher blood pressure, lower high-density lipoprotein (HDL) cholesterol levels and increased dysfunctional, pro-inflammatory HDL.

A similar study examining arterial stiffness, flow-mediated vasodilation of brachial artery, and carotid artery intima-media thickness between patients with autoimmune disease and controls showed signs of increased carotid intima media thickness and impaired flow-mediated vasodilation (FMD) in patients with autoimmune disease.[21] This study included 13 PM patients who on subgroup analysis had similar values of FMD compared to patients with antiphospholipid antibody syndrome, rheumatoid arthritis, and systemic sclerosis.

Laboratory Testing for Cardiac Involvement

Cardiac isoform troponin-I is the most specific biomarker for myocardial involvement in IIM.[10] Troponin isoform T and CK-MB may be elevated in the setting of cardiac injury in IIM patients, however, they are also expressed in regenerating skeletal muscle fibers. These muscle fibers are commonly noted in biopsies from IIM patients, and consequently elevations in troponin T and CK-MB can occur in the absence of specific cardiac injury. Troponin I, however, is only produced in cardiac muscle, not regenerating fibers, and hence remains normal unless there is specific cardiac injury.

Myositis-specific antibodies can predict other organ manifestations in IIM, such a Jo-1 and ILD or anti-TIF1gamma and malignancy and no such strong correlations between autoantibodies and heart disease in myositis have been reported. A study of an Italian population evaluating the anti-MJ antibody in adult PM/DM found the clinical course to be much more benign than other antibodies, with none of the study population developing cardiac or lung involvement.[22]

Cardiac Symptoms and Outcomes

An extensive review article performed by Gupta and colleagues[23] in 2011 searched the entire MEDLINE database from 1977 to 2009 for keywords related to IIM and cardiac involvement leading to a total of 33 articles (case reports or cohort studies) to evaluate cardiac symptoms in a combined prospective cohort of 195 IIM study patients. Twenty-seven patients (13.8%) had systolic murmur, 21 reported dyspnea

(10.8%), 15 reported angina (7.7%), 10 had palpitations, and 3 had peripheral edema. In the same study by Gupta and colleagues, analysis of a 290 patients in retrospective studies revealed 43% of patients reporting combined symptoms of chest pain, dyspnea, and edema. Among the same retrospective study population, CHF was the most common event, occurring in 34 (11.7%) patients followed by arrhythmia in 7 patients. In the prospective cohort, however, arrhythmia was most common at 13.8%, followed by CHF (5.6%) and myocardial infarction (MI) (2.4%).

In the same review article, cardiac causes of death were reported in some of the prospective and retrospective studies. Among 102 prospective patients, 7 died of MI, 4 of CHF, and 4 of myocarditis. Among 550 retrospective patients, 2 died of cardiac arrests, 4 died of arrhythmias, 3 from CHF, 2 from MI, and 3 of third-degree heart block. When combined in total, the authors reported that 51 total had died with CHF (21%) as the leading cause followed by MI (18%).

Another review article investigating cardiac symptoms was conducted by Zhang and colleagues[24] in 2012 based on 26 articles in Medline from 1975 to 2011 that totaled 1530 patients. They observed again that there was a wide range of heart involvement in PM/DM patients between 9% and 72% depending on the authors' methods used to detect cardiac involvement and patient selection. Interestingly, they reported that severity of the muscle findings in IIM patients did not correlate with the presence of cardiac disease in multiple studies. Their review also reported that it is likely that nearly 3% to 6% of all cardiac involvement in IIM is asymptomatic.

Zhang and colleagues[24] found that CHF was the most reported clinical cardiac involvement from 32% to 77% of the patients in the review article. They stated that heart disease could occur during periods of stable or active PM/DM. Reviewing tests including ECG, Holter, and radionuclide ventriculography, they found a rate of 13% to 72% of subclinical heart complications. ST-T changes were the most commonly found ECG abnormality. Left atrial/left ventricular enlargement (8%–12%), LVH (8%–15%), septal hypertrophy (8%), valvular disease (7%–23%), pulmonary hypertension (63%–75%), and pericardial effusion (8–66.7) were also identified.

Regarding mortality outcomes, the review by Zhang found 132 deaths among the 1530 patients, with 37 dying as a direct result of heart disease. In their prospective studies, they found 11 deaths in 78 patients, 9 of which had cardiac complications.

Shu and colleagues[25] from China retrospectively investigated survival among 188 patients at one hospital with IIM from 1986-2009 and showed that 34% of all patients studied had cardiac involvement. Cardiac involvement was found to be a statistically significant risk factor for death ($P = 0.023$) in the non-survival group with 17 of 32 deaths (53.1%) having cardiac involvement, equal to interstitial lung disease. On a Cox regression model and further statistical analysis, however, the authors concluded that neither cardiac nor lung disease were risk factors for mortality which was contrary to other studies.

Both the Gupta and Zhang reviews concluded that IIM patients with cardiac involvement fared worse than those IIM patients without cardiac involvement. They agreed in baseline screening for cardiac symptoms and suggested baseline ECG followed by any other tests if indicated (echocardiography, troponin, etc).

Treatments

Given the limited number of studies regarding cardiac involvement in IIM, it is not surprising that there is even less information regarding formal recommendations for treatment. Specific guidelines for immune suppression as it relates to improving cardiac outcomes are not available. What is clear from the literature is that IIM patients with cardiac involvement are more likely to be hospitalized or die as a result of their cardiac involvement than patients without cardiac involvement. The challenge in IIM patients is to determine whether their cardiac disease is a result of direct muscle inflammation or as a consequence of small-vessel/coronary disease from therapies for IIM (steroids) and prolonged inflammation. It is thought that patients suffering from true inflammatory changes in the heart (monocellular infiltrate into cardiac muscle) directly related to IIM are most likely to respond to immune suppression. In these situations it seems reasonable to give aggressive therapy to control the IIM to prevent long-term damage and remodeling, although large studies are lacking. Some studies have shown improvement with CHF using steroids but other reports showed progression of arrhythmias.[6]

For patients with coronary artery disease, most studies suggest treating underlying traditional risk factors for CAD in IIM patients, such as hypertension and dyslipidemia. When patients do develop sequelae of cardiac damage in the form of CHF, arrhythmia, cardiomyopathy, etc, they are treated similarly to patients without IIM. Medications used commonly for these conditions include β-blockers, ACE inhibitors, and lipid-lowering agents, among others. A special consideration should be made for patients with Raynaud syndrome to evaluate for vasospastic prinzmetal's angina.

Lipid-lowering agents such as HMG-CoA reductase inhibitors (statins) have been associated with marked reduction in CV morbidity and mortality in the general population.[26] Data also suggests potential immunomodulatory effects in patients with rheumatic disease, in particular rheumatoid arthritis.[27] However, in the setting of IIM, concern often exists amongst both clinicians and patients regarding the association of statins with myopathy as a potential adverse effect. New data has also described an auto-immune necrotizing myopathy, which is a rare condition in which myopathy develops and persists after discontinuation of statins, and is associated with specific autoantibody testing.[28,29]

A survey of clinical experts in IIM belonging to the International Myositis Assessment and clinical Studies (IMACS) group evaluated cholesterol-lowering medication use among 1641 IIM patients. Seventy-six percent of these specialists treating adult IIM patients reported using lipid-lowering therapies in their patients.[30] Statins were the most commonly used agents (93%). In more than 300 patients that were prescribed lipid-lowering therapy, there were 36 cases of worsening myositis. Seven of 8 IMACS experts who reported worsening in myositis patients with lipid-lowering therapies reported cases in which the myositis improved after holding therapy. This survey suggests that statins are commonly used by physicians specializing in the treatment of patients with IIM and that some myositis patients worsen with statin use and may improve on dechallenge. More research regarding the safety of lipid-lowering agents in patients with IIM is warranted.

SUMMARY

Systemic autoimmune diseases are becoming increasingly linked to accelerated risks of cardiovascular disease and events. What is apparent from the above review is that the IIM are not an exception to this growing pattern. Although not always clinically apparent, there seems to be a large percentage of patients who have subclinical CV involvement. Many of the traditional risk factors for CAD, such as hypertension and hyperlipidemia, are associated with developing cardiac involvement in patients with IIM. At this time, it is unclear how much of the atherosclerotic CV morbidity and mortality in IIM patients is driven by traditional CV risk factors versus the effects of chronic systemic inflammation from the underlying IIM. The effects of immunosuppression on cardiac disease and events in IIM patients requires further investigation in carefully controlled studies.

IIM patients with cardiac involvement are at increased risk for overall mortality when compared with IIM patients without CV disease. The risk of severe cardiac and vascular disease complications seems to be higher than that of the general population. Treatments can be focused on preventing traditional cardiovascular risk factors including avoidance of corticosteroids when possible, although this task remains challenging in IIM as is true of other rheumatic diseases. Once complications do develop, they should be managed similarly to patients without IIM. The use of statins for hyperlipidemia and atherosclerosis in IIM is an area that is in need of further investigation, although initial work suggests that their use is not uncommon by IIM specialists. Further work is needed to determine whether aggressive immunosuppressive treatment of patients with subclinical cardiac disease will lead to better outcomes. Work is also needed in the area of better laboratory, imaging, and serologic testing to identify patients at risk for the worst cardiovascular complications. At this point, based on the body of evidence reviewed here and elsewhere, it is imperative that physicians treating IIM patients perform a routine cardiovascular risk assessment at the onset of diagnosis. Appropriate diagnostic and monitoring studies should be performed on those patients who screening history or examination is suggestive of cardiac involvement.

REFERENCES

1. Nagaraju K, Lundberg IE. Inflammatory diseases of muscle and other myopathies. 9th edition. Kelleys Textbook of Rheumatology; 2012. p. 1404–30.
2. National Institue of Environmental Health Sciences. International Myositis Assessment and Clinical Research (IMACS) 2011. Available at: http://www.niehs.nih.gov/news/events/pastmtg/imacs/index.cfm.
3. Cruellas MG, Viana Vdos S, Levy-Neto M, et al. Myositis-specific and myositis-associated autoantibody profiles and their clinical associations in large series of patients with polymyositis and dermatomyositis. Clinics 2013;68(7):909–14.
4. Wallace E, Wortmann R. Diagnosis and management of inflammatory muscle disease. J Musculoskelet Med 2001;27:12.
5. Lundberg IE. The heart in dermatomyositis and polymyositis. Rheumatology 2006;45(Suppl 4):iv18–21.
6. Kassi M, Nabi F. Role of Cardiac MRI in the assessment of nonischemic cardiomyopahties. Methodist Debakey Cardiovasc J 2013;9(3):149–55.
7. Mavrogeni S, Douskou M, Manoussakis M. Contrast-enhanced CMR imaging reveals myocardial involvement in idiopathic inflammatory myopathy without cardiac manifestations. JACC Cardiovasc Imaging 2011;4:1324–5.
8. Ponfick M, Gdynia HJ, Kassubek J, et al. Cardiac involvement in juvenile overlap-myositis detected by cardiac magnetic resonance imaging. Int J Cardiol 2011;152:e25–6.
9. Mavrogeni S, Bratis K, Karabela G, et al. Myocarditis during acute inflammatory myopathies-evaluations using clinical criteria and cardiac magnetic resonance imaging. Int J Cardiol 2013;164:e3–4.
10. Sénéchal M, Martin C, Poirier P. Myocardial dysfunction in polymyositis. Can J Cardiol 2006;22(10):869–71.
11. Schwartz T, Sanner H, Husebye T, et al. Cardiac dysfunction in juvenile dermatomyositis: a case-control study. Ann Rheum Dis 2011;70:766–71.
12. Cox F, Delgado V, Vershuuren J, et al. The heart in sporadic inclusion body myositis: a study in 51 patients. J Neurol 2010;257:447–51.
13. Ballo P, Chiodi L, Cameli M, et al. Dilated cardiomyopathy and inclusion body myositis. Neurol Sci 2012;33:367–70.

14. Hollan I, Meroni PL, Ahearn JM, et al. Cardiovascular disease in autoimmune rheumatic diseases. Autoimmun Rev 2013;12(10):1004–15.
15. Linos E, Fiorentino D, Lingala B, et al. Atherosclerotic cardiovascular disease and dermatomyositis: an analysis of the Nationwide Inpatient Sample survey. Arthritis Res Ther 2013;15:R7.
16. Zoller B, Li X, Sundquist J, et al. Risk of subsequent coronary heat disease in patients hospitalized for immune mediated diseases: a nationwide follow-up study from Sweden. PLoS One 2012;7:e33442.
17. Zoller B, Li X, Sundquist J, et al. Risk of subsequent ischemic and hemorrhagic stroke in patients hospitalized for immune-mediated diseases: a nationwide follow up study from Sweden. BMC Neurol 2012;12:41.
18. Tisseverasinghe A, Bernatsky S, Pineau CA. Arterial events in persons with Dermatomyositis and Polymyositis. J Rheumatol 2009;36(9):1943–6.
19. Limaye VS, Lester S, Blumbergs P, et al. Idiopathic inflammatory myositis is associated with a high incidence of hypertension and diabetes mellitus. Int J Rheum Dis 2010;13:132–7.
20. Eimer MJ, Brickman WJ, Seashadri R, et al. Clinical status and cardiovascular risk profile of adults with a history of juvenile dermatomyosits. J Pediatr 2011;159:795–801.
21. Soltész P, Dér H, Kerekes G, et al. A comparative study of arterial stiffness, flow-mediated vasodilation of the brachial artery, and the thickness of the carotid artery intima-media in patients with systemic autoimmune diseases. Clin Rheumatol 2009;28:655–62.
22. Ceribelli A, Fredi M, Taraborelli M, et al. Anti-MJ/NXP-2 autoantibody specificity in a cohort of adult Italian patients with polymyositis/dermatomyositis. Arthritis Res Ther 2012;14(2):R97.
23. Gupta R, Siddharth AW, Ira NT, et al. Clinical cardiac involvement in idiopathic inflammatory myopathies: a systemic review. Int J Cardiol 2011;148:261–70.
24. Zhang L, Wang GC, Ma L, et al. Cardiac involvement in adult polymyositis or dermatomyositis: a systemic review. Clin Cardiol 2012;35(11):686–91.
25. Shu XM, Lu X, Xie Y, et al. Clinical characteristics and favorable long-term outcomes for patients with idiopathic inflammatory myopathies: a retrospective single center study in China. BMC Neurol 2011;11:143.
26. Ridker PM, Danielson E, Fonseca FA, et al. Rosuvastatin to prevent vascular events in men and women with elevated C-reactive protein. N Engl J Med 2008;359(21):2195–207.
27. McCarey DW, McInnes IB, Madhok R, et al. Trial of Atorvastatin in Rheumatoid Arthritis (TARA): double-blind, randomised placebo-controlled trial. Lancet 2004;363(9426):2015–21.
28. Mohassel P, Mammen AL. The spectrum of statin myopathy. Curr Opin Rheumatol 2013;25(6):747–52.
29. Mammen AL, Chung T, Christopher-Stine L, et al. Autoantibodies against 3-hydroxy-3-methylglutaryl-coenzyme A reductase in patients with statin-associated autoimmune myopathy. Arthritis Rheum 2011;63(3):713–21.
30. Charles-Schoeman C, Amjadi SS, Paulus HE. International Myositis and Clinical Studies Group. Treatment of dyslipidemia in idiopathic inflammatory myositis: results of the International Myositis Assessment and Clinical Studies Group Survey. Clin Rheumatol 2012;3(8):1163–8.

The Heart in Vasculitis

Eli Miloslavsky, MD, Sebastian Unizony, MD*

KEYWORDS

- Vasculitis • Takayasu arteritis • Churg-Strauss syndrome • Polyarteritis nodosa
- Heart disease • Cardiomyopathy • Coronary arteritis

KEY POINTS

- Pericarditis, myocarditis, coronary arteritis, and valvular heart disease have variable incidence across all different forms of primary vasculitis.
- Arteritis of the epicardial coronary arteries is more frequent in Takayasu's arteritis, polyarteritis nodosa, and Behcet's disease; however, angiitis of the main coronaries and vasculitis of the myocardial coronary microcirculation have been observed in most primary vasculitides.
- Pathology and cardiac imaging studies have found that cardiac involvement in vasculitis is often subclinical (eg, Takayasu's arteritis, polyarteritis nodosa, eosinophilic granulomatosis with polyangiitis, and Behcet's disease); however, the morbidity and mortality impact of this phenomenon remains unknown.
- With the exception of pericarditis, most cardiac manifestations require aggressive immunosuppression, whereas coronary and valvular disease may also need surgical intervention with revascularization or valve replacement.
- When surgery is indicated, perioperative and long-term control of the inflammation is of paramount importance to assure surgical success and prevent future complications, such as graft and stent restenosis or valvular dehiscence.

INTRODUCTION

Heart involvement in primary systemic vasculitides is important to recognize, because it has been linked to increased mortality and requires prompt diagnosis and treatment. Almost all primary vasculitides can target the heart. Although cardiac compromise is a rare manifestation in vasculitis, with less than 10% of patients affected overall, certain entities, such as eosinophilic granulomatosis with polyangiitis (EGPA, formerly Churg-Strauss syndrome) and Takayasu's arteritis (TAK) can cause heart complications in up to 60% of patients. Any cardiac tissue can be involved, and patients present with varied clinicopathologic syndromes including pericarditis, myocarditis, coronary arteritis,

Rheumatology Unit, Division of Rheumatology, Allergy, and Immunology, Department of Medicine, Massachusetts General Hospital, Yawkey 2, 55 Fruit Street, Boston, MA 02114, USA
* Corresponding author.
E-mail address: sunizony@partners.org

Rheum Dis Clin N Am 40 (2014) 11–26
http://dx.doi.org/10.1016/j.rdc.2013.10.006
0889-857X/14/$ – see front matter © 2014 Elsevier Inc. All rights reserved.

valvulopathy, and intracavitary cardiac thrombosis (**Table 1**). A high index of suspicion is required, because electrocardiography (ECG), echocardiography, cardiac magnetic resonance imaging (cMRI), and coronary angiography are not completely sensitive or specific for diagnosing vasculitic injury, and histologic sampling is not always possible. Therapy depends on the specific manifestation and whether it represents active disease or prior damage (healed or "burnt out" disease). Both medical and surgical management approaches have been described, although controlled studies of treatment outcomes have not yet been carried out in most vasculitides. We herein describe cardiac manifestations of large-, medium-, and small-vessel primary systemic vasculitides in adults as well as their diagnosis and treatment.

LARGE-VESSEL VASCULITIS
Takayasu Arteritis

Cardiac disease is a major cause of morbidity and mortality in TAK.[1–4] Any structure of the heart can potentially be affected, and nearly half of the patients have cardiac involvement at some point during the course of their disease.[5–7] Volume overload (ie, aortic insufficiency), pressure overload (ie, hypertension caused by aortic or renal artery stenosis), myocardial ischemia (ie, coronary arteritis), and myocarditis often lead to left ventricular dysfunction. Other manifestations comprise pericarditis, ischemic heart disease secondary to accelerated atherosclerosis, pulmonary hypertension–induced right heart failure, arrhythmia, and sudden cardiac death. Signs and symptoms reflecting cardiac disease include chest pain, dyspnea, orthopnea, peripheral edema, palpitations, heart murmur, pericardial rub, neck vein distention, lung crackles, and syncope. Although good quality evidence to guide therapy in TAK is lacking, many cardiac manifestations require both medical and surgical interventions.

Aortic insufficiency (AI) is reported in 15% to 50% of TAK patients depending on the diagnostic method used.[3,5–13] This complication occurs primarily as a consequence of annular dilatation and valvular leaflet separation produced in the context of ascending aortitis and aneurysm formation (**Fig. 1**). Less frequently, inflammatory retraction of the aortic valve is the pathogenic mechanism. The clinical presentation of AI ranges from asymptomatic to rapidly progressive congestive heart failure (CHF). An echocardiographic follow-up study of 76 patients with TAK found AI in 40% of the subjects. Valvular regurgitation was mild, moderate, and severe in 71%, 16%, and 13% of these

Table 1
Cardiac manifestations of primary vasculitides

Primary Vasculitis	Pericarditis	Myocarditis	Valvulopathy	Epicardial Coronary Arteries	Coronary Microcirculation	Intracavitary Thrombus
				Coronary Vasculitis		
TAK	X	X	X	X	—	X
GCA	X	X	X	X	—	—
PAN	X	X	—	X	X	—
EGPA	X	X	X	X	X	X
GPA/MPA	X	X	X	X	X	X
CV	X	—	—	X	X	—
BD	X	X	X	X	X	X

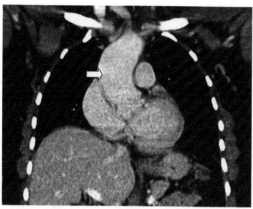

Fig. 1. Computed tomography angiography shows aneurysmal dilatation of the ascending aorta (*arrow*) in a patient with TAK. A subsequent echocardiogram showed moderate aortic insufficiency by color Doppler.

cases, respectively.[10] Mitral and tricuspid valvulopathies, reported in approximately 20% of patients, were typically mild.

According to the severity of the AI (eg, grade, symptomatic burden, and ventricular function impairment), treatment includes aortic valve replacement (AVR), preferably in conjunction with aortic root replacement, and immunosuppression depending on disease activity.[14] When possible, elective surgical interventions should be performed when TAK is judged to be quiescent. In the face of active disease, clinical judgment is important to weight the risks and benefits of delaying surgery until immunosuppression takes effect versus operating in an inflammatory milieu. Although corticosteroids (CS) may affect wound healing, cardiovascular surgeons generally agree with the judicious use of these agents in the perioperative period to adequately control vascular inflammation and prevent dehiscence of the prosthetic valve or pseudoaneurysmal formation at the suture line.[15]

Coronary artery involvement is demonstrated by angiography in up to 60% of the patients, but becomes symptomatic in 5% to 20% of the cases.[1,3,5,7,9,10,16] Patients present with angina, acute myocardial infarction, arrhythmia, conduction abnormalities, or CHF. Along with aortic valve disease, myocardial ischemia is a leading cause of death in TAK.[2] Stenosis and occlusions tend to occur in the coronary ostia (>70%) and proximal segments (**Fig. 2**). Less frequently, diffuse or focal distal narrowing, coronary aneurysms, and intercoronary or coronary-bronchial artery fistulizations are seen.[12,17,18] Vascular inflammation is the main mechanism of coronary arteriopathy. Ostial obstructions are often caused by the extension of the adjacent aortic process (ie, intimal proliferation and fibrotic retraction). However, premature atherosclerosis secondary to hypertension and a chronic inflammatory state is an important adjuvant factor.[19] Except in rare cases (ie, string of pearls pattern of arterial stenoses and dilatations), the angiographic features do not entirely define the inflammatory or noninflammatory nature of coronary lesions in TAK. The diagnosis of coronary vasculitis often requires high clinical suspicion and the integration of data from multiple sources (eg, extracardiac manifestations, level of inflammatory markers, evidence of active large vessel involvement in cross sectional vascular imaging).

The treatment of coronary artery disease in TAK has medical and surgical implications. CS in combination with other immunosuppressive agents are indicated when active vasculitis is presumed to be the cause. When revascularization is required, consultation

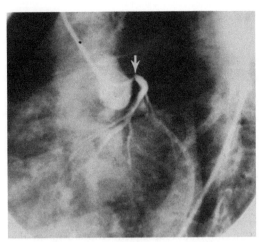

Fig. 2. Coronary angiogram shows a stenotic lesion involving the ostium of the left coronary artery (*arrow*) in a patient with TAK. (*Courtesy of* Dr Michael Jaff, Boston, MA.)

with an experienced cardiovascular surgeon is mandatory. Coronary artery bypass grafting (CABG), balloon angioplasty followed by stenting, and transaortic endarterectomy are used depending on the number, location, and characteristics of the lesions.[18] Proximal stenoses are frequently bypassed with a large-diameter, aorto-coronary, saphenous vein graft. Surgical treatment should be avoided, when possible, during periods of active inflammation. In situ internal thoracic artery CABG is often not recommended given the frequent vasculitic involvement of the subclavian arteries (40%–80%).[20] The incidence of restenosis within 5 to 10 years after the procedure is significantly higher after angioplasty with stent placement than after bypass surgery (10%–80% vs 5%–40%).[7,8] Case reports suggest that drug-eluting stents (ie, sirolimus) may decrease (or delay) the occurrence of this complication. In all cases, adequate control of disease activity is fundamental for long-term maintenance of graft and stent patency.[21,22]

The possibility of myocarditis should be entertained when a patient with TAK presents with chest pain or heart failure in the absence of pericardial, coronary, or valvular lesions. Laboratory workup may find elevated cardiac biomarkers, and echocardiogram frequently shows left ventricular hypokinesis and dilatation (ie, dilated cardiomyopathy).[23,24] Although cMRI may discover myocardial damage (ie, late gadolinium enhancement),[13] endomyocardial biopsy is the gold standard for diagnosis. Histologic features include myocyte necrosis, myocytolysis, and interstitial foci of mononuclear inflammatory cells (mainly lymphocytes, natural killer cells, and histiocytes).[24,25] Some studies indicate that up to 50% of the patients with TAK have some degree of myocardial inflammation, which is often subclinical.[24,26] Increased expression of perforins and major histocompatibility complex molecules within the inflammatory lesions point toward cell-mediated cytotoxicity as one of the injury mechanisms.[27] Myocarditis treatment requires immunosuppression (eg, prednisone and cyclophosphamide) combined with conventional heart failure therapy (eg, diuretics).[25,27] Secondary cardiomyopathy can occur in the setting of chronic hypertension (seen in approximately 70% of TAK patients),[10,12] valvulopathy, and ischemic coronary disease. In these situations, correction of the underlying cause (eg, renal artery stenting, AVR, or coronary revascularization) and aggressive specific therapy (eg, β-blockers, angiotensin-converting enzyme inhibitors) is essential, as CHF is a risk factor for poor prognosis in this disorder.[3,12]

The pulmonary arteries are affected in up to 50% of TAK patients. However, clinically significant pulmonary arterial hypertension (PAH; World Health Organization [WHO] class 1) is seen in about a quarter of these cases.[3,5,6,12] In other instances, postcapillary pulmonary hypertension (WHO class 2) complicates left heart disease (eg, AI or hypertensive cardiomyopathy). Arterial or venous pulmonary hypertension is generally mild to moderate, therefore, rarely leads to right ventricular failure.[28]

Pericarditis occurs in about 8% of the subjects with TAK,[7] generally as part of a febrile syndrome, and sometimes as the initial manifestation of the disease.[29] Treatment of pericardial inflammation includes nonsteroidal anti-inflammatory drugs (NSAIDs) or moderate doses of CS.

Giant Cell Arteritis

The incidence of heart involvement by giant cell arteritis (GCA) is low (<5%), but rigorous studies addressing this problem are lacking. As in TAK, disease-specific cardiac manifestations of GCA encompass pericarditis, coronary vasculitis, myocarditis, and aortic regurgitation caused by ascending aortic aneurysm.

Coronary arteritis is a rare but potentially fatal complication of GCA.[30–33] Patients may present with chest pain, dyspnea, CHF, arrhythmia, and sudden cardiac death. Concomitant cardiovascular risk factors, commonly present in this elderly population, make the differentiation between vasculitis- and atherosclerosis-induced coronary artery disease challenging.[34] Unfortunately, serologic (ie, cardiac enzymes), ECG, and angiographic features are not pathognomonic. Therefore, recognition of coronary vasculitis in this setting demands a high index of suspicion.[35] In this regard, concurrent cranial symptoms or polymyalgia rheumatica in a GCA patient presenting with acute coronary syndrome may suggest active vasculitis and prompt the administration of high-dose prednisone in addition to treatment of myocardial ischemia (eg, antiplatelet therapy, statins, anticoagulation, revascularization). As in TAK, the use of in situ internal thoracic artery grafts for coronary revascularization is not advised in GCA, because the subclavian arteries are affected in 40% to 75% of the patients.[20,36] Paradoxically, acute myocardial infarction soon after the initiation of CS for otherwise classic GCA has been occasionally reported, but the significance of this rare phenomenon remains unclear.[31,37]

Exudative pericarditis is unusual in GCA.[38,39] Patients tend to present with pleuritic chest pain, dyspnea, and friction rubs along with other evidence of active disease (ie, cranial symptoms or polymyalgia rheumatica). However, up to 30% of the cases described occurred in the absence of concomitant typical GCA manifestations. At any rate, excluding malignancy, infection, drug reactions, endocrine, and metabolic disorders is important before assuming that GCA is the cause of a pericardial effusion in the elderly.

Documentation of myocarditis in GCA is limited to isolated case reports.[40–42] Clinical presentation mimics that of coronary vasculitis, as patients present with chest pain, ECG changes, and elevated cardiac enzymes. Cardiac MRI with contrast enhancement may represent a useful noninvasive diagnostic modality.[42] However, histologic confirmation, which shows lymphohistiocytic inflammation with or without giant cells, is sometimes required.[40]

MEDIUM-VESSEL VASCULITIS
Polyarteritis Nodosa

Clinically apparent heart involvement occurs in 5% to 20% of patients with polyarteritis nodosa (PAN).[43–46] Inflammatory cardiac manifestations include coronary arteritis, fibrinous pericarditis, and, rarely, myocarditis.[47,48] As the end result of myocardial ischemia, or in the setting of severe hypertension (ie, vasculitic renal artery stenosis), these patients may also have left ventricular dysfunction.[48] Acute myocardial infarction and CHF are serious complications of PAN with prognostic implications (ie, five factor score [FFS]).[48–51]

Chest pain, electrocardiographic ischemic changes, troponin elevation, and variable degrees of ventricular wall motion abnormalities are presenting manifestations of coronary arteritis in PAN.[48,52,53] In the setting of ischemia, patients can also have rhythm and conduction defects, including sudden cardiac death.[54] Autopsy studies have found inflammation of the main coronary arteries and their proximal branches in 40% to 50% of the patients[48,55] and vasculitis limited to the small myocardial arterioles (without involvement of the epicardial coronary vessels) in 25% of the cases.[48] In these reports, only 4 of 102 cases were clinically diagnosed as acute myocardial infarction antemortem. However, 60% to 70% of the examined hearts had signs of prior ischemic injury.[48,55]

In established PAN lesions, fibrinoid necrosis in association with acute and chronic inflammatory infiltrates and fibrosis (depending on the stage of the process) may produce mural-thickening, luminal stenosis, superimposed thrombosis, dissection, or aneurysmal dilatations. Therefore, coronary angiography may not only show focal or diffuse areas of narrowing and occlusion but also the characteristic pattern of "beads on a string" as seen in other vascular territories (ie, mesenteric vessels).[47,51–53] In cases of isolated microvascular disease, angiography may be totally normal. As in other forms of vasculitis (see TAK and GCA), the differentiation of inflammatory and atherosclerotic coronary artery disease is often challenging, and good clinical judgment is of prime importance. At times, a mesenteric angiogram or a nerve and/or muscle biopsy can be the test that defines the underlying diagnosis.[47,52] Coronary arteritis requires aggressive immunosuppression (ie, high doses of CS and cyclophosphamide)[56] and often revascularization. Anecdotal evidence describes successful use of saphenous vein as well as internal thoracic artery grafts for CABG. When implementing the latter strategy, previous angiographic evaluation of the internal thoracic artery is recommended to rule out vasculitic stenosis or occlusion.[57,58]

Coronary angiitis and hypertension are the main pathogenic mechanisms that lead to cardiac failure in PAN. The hearts of these individuals often have myocardiocyte hypertrophy and scarring from prior ischemic insults.[48] In a series of 348 well-characterized patients, the incidence of severe hypertension and vasculitis-related cardiomyopathy was 6.9% and 7.5%, respectively. These complications were significantly more frequent in hepatitis B virus (HBV)-related PAN (approximately 10%).[46] Cardiac causes (ie, myocardial infarction and sudden cardiac death) explained 3.5% of the 5-year mortality in this cohort. In another study, which included many of the above-mentioned research subjects, cardiomyopathy was associated with a higher risk of death (hazard ratio of 2.47 and 3.54 for non–HBV-related PAN and HBV-related PAN, respectively).[59]

The management of PAN-induced cardiomyopathy includes immunosuppressive therapy for patients with active vasculitis and antiviral agents for subjects with ongoing HBV infection. Hypertension and heart failure should be aggressively treated in PAN as in any other clinical scenario. Careful evaluation of the renal arteries is mandatory for the identification of renal artery stenosis that may require angioplastic correction.

Nonuremic acute fibrinous pericarditis has been reported in 5% to 10% of the patients with PAN. Myocarditis is rare and usually mild.[46,48,55]

SMALL-VESSEL VASCULITIS
Eosinophilic Granulomatosis with Polyangiitis

Cardiac involvement in EGPA is common and often severe.[49,50,60–62] The importance of recognizing heart disease in EGPA cannot be underestimated because the presence of cardiomyopathy has been shown to be the most important predictor of mortality in this population.[63]

Cardiac involvement in EGPA occurs in 15% to 60% of cases.[60,61,63–70] The most frequent manifestations are pericarditis and cardiomyopathy, each occurring in approximately 15% to 30% of patients. Valvular lesions, detected in up to 30%, are frequently asymptomatic.[66] In addition, coronary vasculitis and heart block are seen in less than 3% of the individuals, whereas intraventricular thrombus formation is limited to isolated reports.[71] The most common clinical symptoms include those of arrhythmia and heart failure. Angina is less frequently seen. Although cardiovascular involvement is usually an early manifestation, it can also occur later in the course of the disease.[60,64,66] Patients with cardiac disease tend to be antineutrophil cytoplasmic antibody negative, have higher eosinophil counts, and experience a shorter delay from the onset of symptoms to definite diagnosis than those without heart compromise.[61,63,66,68]

Noncardiac manifestations of EGPA in patients with cardiac involvement do not differ significantly from those in subjects without heart disease.[66] More than 90% of the cases have asthma at the time of diagnosis, with the remainder of patients having otorhinolaryngologic abnormalities, including sinusitis, rhinitis, and nasal polyposis. Constitutional symptoms, peripheral neuropathy, lung infiltrates, and skin, gastrointestinal, or renal compromise typically coexist with cardiac involvement. However, isolated eosinophilic coronary arteritis in the absence of other features of EGPA has been described.[72–75] It is unclear whether this entity represents a variant of single-organ vasculitis or a limited form of EGPA.

The diagnosis of EGPA-induced heart disease can be challenging, because a significant proportion of patients with cardiac involvement are asymptomatic.[67] Dennert and colleagues[66] found that of 32 patients with EGPA in apparent clinical remission and without prior cardiac manifestations, more than 60% had ECG, echocardiography, or cMRI abnormalities. ECG changes were noted in 66%, echocardiographic defects in 50%, and cMRI abnormalities in 62%. Notably, all 3 diagnostic modalities were not completely sensitive for detecting cardiac involvement. Echocardiography was 83% sensitive compared with cMRI, and cMRI was 88% sensitive compared with echocardiography. Moreover, in the absence of symptoms or major ECG abnormalities, cardiac disease was detected in 40% of patients, leading the authors to conclude that the evaluation for heart involvement in patients with EGPA should include both ECG and cardiac imaging with echocardiography or cMRI. Neumann and colleagues[65] had similar findings, with 23% of patients with confirmed cardiac lesions having normal ECGs and 10% having normal echocardiograms.

Cardiac MRI may be particularly useful in differentiating EGPA myocarditis from other causes of myocardial injury. Delayed contrast enhancement on cMRI has been associated with active myocarditis or endomyocardial fibrosis.[76] Although endomyocardial fibrosis can be seen after ischemic injury as well, the pattern of involvement in myocarditis is not restricted to a specific vascular territory as is seen in patients with coronary artery disease. Finally, the location of ventricular enhancement can also offer a clue to the underlying diagnosis. For example, myocardial inflammation in EGPA and other hypereosinophilic disorders is primarily seen in the apical and midcavity segments, compared with sarcoidosis, in which late gadolinium uptake is seen primarily in the basal segments, or acute myocarditis, in which subepicardial and midmyocardial segments are most affected.[66,77] Other studies suggest that positron emission tomography may also have a role for the diagnosis of myocarditis in these subjects.[78,79]

Myocardial injury in EGPA is mainly caused by eosinophilic cytotoxicity, as the histologic picture seen in this disease is similar to the one observed in other hypereosinophilic syndromes (HES).[80] Microscopic examination of the cardiac tissue reveals endomyocardial fibrosis, myocardial lymphocytic infiltration, and marked eosinophilia.[66] Immunohistochemistry staining shows the presence of eosinophil-derived cationic proteins (ie, major basic protein) within the inflammatory lesions.[81,82] In contrast, vasculitis, which is often a hallmark of EGPA in other organs (as opposed to HES), is rarely seen in the myocardium. Despite patchy involvement, cardiac biopsy has been reported to have sensitivity as high as 89%,[63] although large series of patients undergoing tissue sampling are lacking.

Given the considerable mortality associated with cardiac involvement in EGPA, up to 83% of deaths in one series,[64] those with an FFS $\geq$1 should be treated with CS and an additional immunosuppressant, most commonly cyclophosphamide.[60,83] Immunosuppressive treatment has been associated with improvement in arrhythmias and cardiac function.[66] Patients with isolated pericarditis and no other major organ involvement can be treated with CS monotherapy, although more than 50% will require additional immunosuppression during the course of their disease.[63,84]

Granulomatosis with Polyangiitis and Microscopic Polyangiitis

In contrast to EGPA, symptomatic heart involvement is seen in a small percentage of patients with granulomatosis with polyangiitis (GPA; formerly Wegener's granulomatosis). Pericarditis and arrhythmias are the most common cardiac manifestations, occurring in 1% to 6% of patients. Arrhythmias tend to be supraventricular and are hypothesized to occur as a result of sinus node dysfunction, which may be secondary to pericardial inflammation.[85] Involvement of the conduction system structures is uncommon, although atrioventricular block has been reported.[86] Myocarditis, coronary arteritis, and cardiac thrombus are less frequent manifestations, each occurring in less than 1% to 2% of patients.[87–89] Valvular lesions (mainly aortic) are rare, with approximately 20 cases described in the English-language medical literature to date.[90] Mechanisms of valve disruption include valvular masses, some mimicking endocarditis, and valve thickening. Intracardiac atrial and ventricular masses are also uncommon and are limited to case reports.[91]

Subclinical cardiac involvement however may be much more frequent. In a classic clinicopathologic study, Walton[92] observed focal cardiac vasculitis in 28% of patients and intracardiac granulomas in 11%. In an echocardiographic study of patients with GPA, 31% were found to have abnormalities attributable to vasculitis or granulomatosis. Of these, wall motion defects were seen in 65% of patients, decreased left ventricular ejection fraction in 50%, pericardial effusions in 19%, and valvular lesions in 15%.[93]

Research on cardiac involvement in microscopic polyangiitis (MPA) remains limited. A case series reported evidence of heart failure in 18% of patients and pericarditis in 11% among 85 subjects with MPA.[94] Cardiomyopathy was noted in 11% of patients in another large series.[64] Despite these reports, severe heart failure and valvular disease are rare. As in other vasculitides, subclinical disease might be more frequent than clinically apparent disease, but studies addressing this issue are lacking.

Cryoglobulinemic Vasculitis

Cardiac manifestations are reported in 4%–8% of patients with cryoglobulinemic vasculitis (CV).[95,96] Pericarditis, myocardial ischemia, and acute CHF, the usual presenting syndromes, are caused by immune complex–mediated vasculitis.[97] Heart compromise typically occurs concomitantly with other severe organ manifestations (eg, kidney or gastrointestinal). Fluid overload and severe hypertension caused by CV-induced glomerulonephritis are often superimposed myocardial stressors. Workup shows increased troponins and natriuretic peptides, electrocardiographic ST-T changes, and echocardiographic ventricular dysfunction. Depending on the blood vessel size affected, angiography may find stenosis or aneurysms of the main coronary arteries and proximal branches or, more frequently, no abnormalities (ie, coronary microcirculation). Treatment, often in an intensive care unit setting given the severity of heart involvement in CV, consists of antivirals (ie, in HCV-associated cases), immunosuppression (eg, prednisone and cyclophosphamide or rituximab), organ support, and adequate management of the pump failure and cardiac ischemia.[98] Some patients have received plasma exchange. Despite a favorable early response, CV patients with cardiac disease have a mortality rate of 50% within 2 years.[95]

VARIABLE-SIZE VASCULITIS
Behcet's Disease

The largest series to date demonstrated cardiac involvement in approximately 6% of individuals with Behcet's disease (BD).[99] Pericarditis was the most common manifestation (39%), followed by valvular lesions (27%, mainly aortic), and myocardial infarction caused by coronary vasculitis (17%). In addition, some patients had myocarditis **(Fig. 3)**. Interestingly, intraventricular thrombosis, a relatively rare cardiac manifestation of vasculitis, was reported in 19% of patients with BD affecting the heart, reflecting the unique predilection for thrombotic complications in this disorder. Notably, cardiac symptoms were the presenting manifestation of BD in one-third of these patients, but ECG finding were frequently normal. Subjects with cardiac disease were more frequently men and were less likely to be HLA-B51 positive.[99] Like in other systemic vasculitides, subclinical cardiac involvement is thought to be prevalent.

As in TAK, PAN, CV, and EGPA, cardiac compromise in BD is associated with increased mortality. Treatment of cardiac manifestations includes aspirin, NSAIDs, and colchicine for pericardial disease and high doses of CS for myocarditis. Coronary vasculitis and significant valvular lesions may require revascularization and surgical valve replacement, respectively, in association with perioperative immunosuppression.

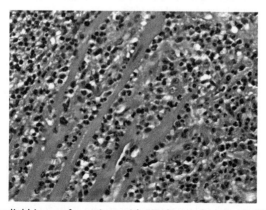

Fig. 3. Endomyocardial biopsy of a patient with BD shows abundant infiltrates of mononuclear inflammatory cells, neutrophils, and eosinophils in between cardiac muscle cells (hematoxylin-eosin, original magnification × 200). (*Courtesy of* Dr James Stone, Boston, MA.)

It should be noted that intraventricular thrombosis in BD may require a combination of surgery, anticoagulation, and immunosuppression, given observed recurrence of clotting with any of those treatment modalities alone.[99–101]

SUMMARY

All primary vasculitides can target the heart, but this complication is more frequent in TAK, PAN, and EGPA. Although pericarditis is seen in virtually all forms of vasculitis, it rarely becomes a significant clinical problem. Myocarditis is more prevalent in EGPA and TAK, and coronary angiitis is most common in TAK, PAN, and BD. In addition, AI is a classic complication of TAK-induced aortitis, and intracavitary cardiac thrombus formation mainly affects patients with BD. Myocarditis, coronary arteritis, and valvular disease can lead to congestive heart failure and represent poor prognostic factors that require aggressive therapy. Imaging and pathology studies have found that subclinical involvement is common (eg, TAK, PAN, EGPA, GPA, and BD). Management differs depending on the cardiac structure involved and the activity of the disease. Although pericarditis can be treated with NSAIDs, colchicine, or-low dose prednisone, myocarditis and coronary vasculitis require high doses of CS and frequently cytotoxic agents. Valvular lesions, coronary arteriopathy, and ventricular thrombosis often need surgical intervention. In the face of active disease, clinical judgment is important to help weigh the risks and benefits of delaying surgery versus operating in possibly inflamed tissues. As in other rheumatic diseases, risks factors for atherosclerosis (eg, hypertension, dyslipidemia) should be identified and corrected. Finally, heart failure– and ischemia-targeted therapies are important components of the treatment strategy when indicated.

Below is a summary of key points

TAK

o Aortitis often leads to ascending aortic aneurysm and AI. Subjects with active disease require immunosuppressive therapy. When AI is symptomatic or causes left ventricular dysfunction, surgical valve replacement is also indicated.

o Symptomatic coronary vasculitis is seen in 5% to 20% of the patients. Treatment often includes aggressive immunosuppression and revascularization. The use of in situ internal thoracic artery bypass grafting is not routinely recommended given the high prevalence of subclavian involvement in large-vessel vasculitis.

o Myocarditis can lead to dilated cardiomyopathy. Other causes of myocardial dysfunction in this population include hypertension, valvular disease, and inflammatory or atherosclerotic coronary arteriopathy.

GCA

o Heart involvement is rare. However, coronary angiitis should be considered in patients presenting with acute coronary syndrome, and aortitis should be suspected in those who have ascending aortic aneurysm and AI.

PAN

o Clinically apparent heart involvement is seen in 5% to 20% of patients. The principal cardiac manifestations include coronary vasculitis and pericarditis. Whereas pericardial disease may resolve with NSAIDs or moderate doses of prednisone, coronary vasculitis portends a poor prognosis and should be treated with high doses of corticosteroids and cyclophosphamide.

o Patients with vasculitic-induced renal artery stenosis are at risk for developing hypertensive cardiomyopathy. Correction of the renovascular hypertension is essential to prevent myocardial damage.

EGPA

○ Myocarditis is seen in 30% of patients and predicts poor prognosis.

○ As in other vasculitides, heart involvement is often subclinical.

○ ECG lacks sensitivity for detecting cardiac disease and echocardiography or cardiac MRI is recommended for screening and diagnosis.

○ Eosinophil-induced damage is the mechanism of myocardial injury. Treatment requires high doses of CS, often in association with cytotoxic agents (ie, cyclophosphamide).

GPA

○ Pericarditis and arrhythmias are the most common cardiac manifestations, occurring in up to 6% of patients. Valvular lesions are rare but can sometimes mimic bacterial endocarditis.

CV

○ Cardiac manifestations such as pericarditis and coronary vasculitis are seen in 4% to 8% of patients. Heart vasculitis may affect the main coronary arteries and the coronary microcirculation and typically occurs concomitantly with other severe organ involvement. In this scenario, high doses of CS in combination with cyclophosphamide or rituximab should be considered.

BD

○ Cardiac disease is seen in approximately 6% of patients. Pericarditis, coronary vasculitis, myocarditis, and intracavitary thrombus formation are the main manifestations. Treatment of thrombosis in BD may not only require anticoagulation and surgery but also immunosuppression to prevent recurrence.

REFERENCES

1. Park MC, Lee SW, Park YB, et al. Clinical characteristics and outcomes of Takayasu's arteritis: analysis of 108 patients using standardized criteria for diagnosis, activity assessment, and angiographic classification. Scand J Rheumatol 2005;34:284–92.
2. Soto ME, Espinola N, Flores-Suarez LF, et al. Takayasu arteritis: clinical features in 110 Mexican Mestizo patients and cardiovascular impact on survival and prognosis. Clin Exp Rheumatol 2008;26:S9–15.
3. Cong XL, Dai SM, Feng X, et al. Takayasu's arteritis: clinical features and outcomes of 125 patients in China. Clin Rheumatol 2010;29:973–81.
4. Numano F. Differences in clinical presentation and outcome in different countries for Takayasu's arteritis. Curr Opin Rheumatol 1997;9:12–5.
5. Kerr GS, Hallahan CW, Giordano J, et al. Takayasu arteritis. Ann Intern Med 1994;120:919–29.
6. Bicakcigil M, Aksu K, Kamali S, et al. Takayasu's arteritis in Turkey - clinical and angiographic features of 248 patients. Clin Exp Rheumatol 2009;27:S59–64.
7. Maksimowicz-McKinnon K, Clark TM, Hoffman GS. Limitations of therapy and a guarded prognosis in an American cohort of Takayasu arteritis patients. Arthritis Rheum 2007;56:1000–9.
8. Ohigashi H, Haraguchi G, Konishi M, et al. Improved prognosis of Takayasu arteritis over the past decade–comprehensive analysis of 106 patients. Circ J 2012;76:1004–11.
9. Lee GY, Jang SY, Ko SM, et al. Cardiovascular manifestations of Takayasu arteritis and their relationship to the disease activity: analysis of 204 Korean patients at a single center. Int J Cardiol 2012;159:14–20.

10. Soto ME, Espinola-Zavaleta N, Ramirez-Quito O, et al. Echocardiographic follow-up of patients with Takayasu's arteritis: five-year survival. Echocardiography 2006;23:353–60.
11. Hashimoto Y, Oniki T, Aerbajinai W, et al. Aortic regurgitation in patients with Takayasu arteritis: assessment by color Doppler echocardiography. Heart Vessels Suppl 1992;7:111–5.
12. Panja M, Kar AK, Dutta AL, et al. Cardiac involvement in non-specific aortoarteritis. Int J Cardiol 1992;34:289–95.
13. Keenan NG, Mason JC, Maceira A, et al. Integrated cardiac and vascular assessment in Takayasu arteritis by cardiovascular magnetic resonance. Arthritis Rheum 2009;60:3501–9.
14. Ando M, Kosakai Y, Okita Y, et al. Surgical treatment for aortic regurgitation caused by Takayasu's arteritis. J Card Surg 1998;13:202–7.
15. Matsuura K, Ogino H, Kobayashi J, et al. Surgical treatment of aortic regurgitation due to Takayasu arteritis: long-term morbidity and mortality. Circulation 2005;112:3707–12.
16. Panja M, Sarkar C, Kar AK, et al. Coronary artery lesions in Takayasu's arteritis–clinical and angiographic study. J Assoc Physicians India 1998;46:678–81.
17. Amano J, Suzuki A. Coronary artery involvement in Takayasu's arteritis. Collective review and guideline for surgical treatment. J Thorac Cardiovasc Surg 1991;102:554–60.
18. Endo M, Tomizawa Y, Nishida H, et al. Angiographic findings and surgical treatments of coronary artery involvement in Takayasu arteritis. J Thorac Cardiovasc Surg 2003;125:570–7.
19. Seyahi E, Ugurlu S, Cumali R, et al. Atherosclerosis in Takayasu arteritis. Ann Rheum Dis 2006;65:1202–7.
20. Grayson PC, Maksimowicz-McKinnon K, Clark TM, et al. Distribution of arterial lesions in Takayasu's arteritis and giant cell arteritis. Ann Rheum Dis 2012;71:1329–34.
21. Fields CE, Bower TC, Cooper LT, et al. Takayasu's arteritis: operative results and influence of disease activity. J Vasc Surg 2006;43:64–71.
22. Park MC, Lee SW, Park YB, et al. Post-interventional immunosuppressive treatment and vascular restenosis in Takayasu's arteritis. Rheumatology (Oxford) 2006;45:600–5.
23. Ghosh S, Sinha DP, Mitra D, et al. Dilated cardiomyopathy in non-specific aortoarteritis. Indian Heart J 1999;51:527–31.
24. Talwar KK, Kumar K, Chopra P, et al. Cardiac involvement in nonspecific aortoarteritis (Takayasu's arteritis). Am Heart J 1991;122:1666–70.
25. Talwar KK, Chopra P, Narula J, et al. Myocardial involvement and its response to immunosuppressive therapy in nonspecific aortoarteritis (Takayasu's disease)–a study by endomyocardial biopsy. Int J Cardiol 1988;21:323–34.
26. Sharma BK, Jain S, Radotra BD. An autopsy study of Takayasu arteritis in India. Int J Cardiol 1998;66(Suppl 1):S85–90 [discussion: S1].
27. Takeda N, Takahashi T, Seko Y, et al. Takayasu myocarditis mediated by cytotoxic T lymphocytes. Intern Med 2005;44:256–60.
28. Kumar S, Moorthy N, Kapoor A. Takayasu's arteritis mimicking unilateral pulmonary artery agenesis in a child with severe pulmonary hypertension and right heart failure: a diagnostic dilemma. Pediatr Cardiol 2011;32:993–7.
29. Fateh-Moghadam S, Huehns S, Schmidt WA, et al. Pericardial effusion as primary manifestation of Takayasu arteritis. Int J Cardiol 2010;145:e33–5.

30. Lie JT. Aortic and extracranial large vessel giant cell arteritis: a review of 72 cases with histopathologic documentation. Semin Arthritis Rheum 1995;24: 422–31.
31. Save-Soderbergh J, Malmvall BE, Andersson R, et al. Giant cell arteritis as a cause of death. Report of nine cases. JAMA 1986;255:493–6.
32. Paulley JW. Ischaemic heart disease in giant cell arteritis. Lancet 1980;1:421.
33. Karger B, Fechner G. Sudden death due to giant cell coronary arteritis. Int J Legal Med 2006;120:377–9.
34. Unizony S, Arias-Urdaneta L, Miloslavsky E, et al. Tocilizumab for the treatment of large-vessel vasculitis (giant cell arteritis, Takayasu arteritis) and polymyalgia rheumatica. Arthritis Care Res (Hoboken) 2012;64:1720–9.
35. How J, Strachan RW, Bewsher PD. Giant cell arteritis–a cardiological blind spot? Am Heart J 1980;100:405–7.
36. Blockmans D, de Ceuninck L, Vanderschueren S, et al. Repetitive 18F-fluoro-deoxyglucose positron emission tomography in giant cell arteritis: a prospective study of 35 patients. Arthritis Rheum 2006;55:131–7.
37. Morris CR, Scheib JS. Fatal myocardial infarction resulting from coronary arteritis in a patient with polymyalgia rheumatica and biopsy-proved temporal arteritis. A case report and review of the literature. Arch Intern Med 1994;154: 1158–60.
38. Bablekos GD, Michaelides SA, Karachalios GN, et al. Pericardial involvement as an atypical manifestation of giant cell arteritis: report of a clinical case and literature review. Am J Med Sci 2006;332:198–204.
39. Matsue Y, Ohno M, Nagahori W, et al. A case of giant cell arteritis with massive pericardial effusion. Heart Vessels 2011;26:562–4.
40. Kennedy LJ Jr, Mitchinson MJ. Giant cell arteritis with myositis and myocarditis. Calif Med 1971;115:84–7.
41. Pugnet G, Pathak A, Dumonteil N, et al. Giant cell arteritis as a cause of acute myocarditis in the elderly. J Rheumatol 2011;38:2497.
42. Daumas A, Rossi P, Jacquier A, et al. Myopericarditis revealing giant cell arteritis in the elderly. J Rheumatol 2012;39:665–6.
43. Cohen RD, Conn DL, Ilstrup DM. Clinical features, prognosis, and response to treatment in polyarteritis. Mayo Clin Proc 1980;55:146–55.
44. Fortin PR, Larson MG, Watters AK, et al. Prognostic factors in systemic necrotizing vasculitis of the polyarteritis nodosa group–a review of 45 cases. J Rheumatol 1995;22:78–84.
45. Guillevin L, Lhote F, Cohen P, et al. Polyarteritis nodosa related to hepatitis B virus. A prospective study with long-term observation of 41 patients. Medicine (Baltimore) 1995;74:238–53.
46. Pagnoux C, Seror R, Henegar C, et al. Clinical features and outcomes in 348 patients with polyarteritis nodosa: a systematic retrospective study of patients diagnosed between 1963 and 2005 and entered into the French Vasculitis Study Group Database. Arthritis Rheum 2010;62:616–26.
47. Przybojewski JZ. Polyarteritis nodosa in the adult. Report of a case with repeated myocardial infarction and a review of cardiac involvement. S Afr Med J 1981;60:512–8.
48. Holsinger DR, Osmundson PJ, Edwards JE. The heart in periarteritis nodosa. Circulation 1962;25:610–8.
49. Guillevin L, Lhote F, Gayraud M, et al. Prognostic factors in polyarteritis nodosa and Churg-Strauss syndrome. A prospective study in 342 patients. Medicine (Baltimore) 1996;75:17–28.

50. Gayraud M, Guillevin L, le Toumelin P, et al. Long-term followup of polyarteritis nodosa, microscopic polyangiitis, and Churg-Strauss syndrome: analysis of four prospective trials including 278 patients. Arthritis Rheum 2001;44:666–75.
51. Brooks MJ, Iyer R. Images in clinical medicine. Coronary arteritis. N Engl J Med 2012;367:658.
52. Chu KH, Menapace FJ, Blankenship JC, et al. Polyarteritis nodosa presenting as acute myocardial infarction with coronary dissection. Cathet Cardiovasc Diagn 1998;44:320–4.
53. McWilliams ET, Khonizy W, Jameel A. Polyarteritis nodosa presenting as acute myocardial infarction in a young man: importance of invasive angiography. Heart 2013;99:1219.
54. Shields LB, Burge M, Hunsaker JC 3rd. Sudden death due to polyarteritis nodosa. Forensic Sci Med Pathol 2012;8:290–5.
55. Schrader ML, Hochman JS, Bulkley BH. The heart in polyarteritis nodosa: a clinicopathologic study. Am Heart J 1985;109:1353–9.
56. Guillevin L, Lhote F, Cohen P, et al. Corticosteroids plus pulse cyclophosphamide and plasma exchanges versus corticosteroids plus pulse cyclophosphamide alone in the treatment of polyarteritis nodosa and Churg-Strauss syndrome patients with factors predicting poor prognosis. A prospective, randomized trial in sixty-two patients. Arthritis Rheum 1995;38:1638–45.
57. Yanagawa B, Kumar P, Tsuneyoshi H, et al. Coronary artery bypass in the context of polyarteritis nodosa. Ann Thorac Surg 2010;89:623–5.
58. Trueb RM, Scheidegger EP, Pericin M, et al. Periarteritis nodosa presenting as a breast lesion: report of a case and review of the literature. Br J Dermatol 1999; 141:1117–21.
59. Bourgarit A, Le Toumelin P, Pagnoux C, et al. Deaths occurring during the first year after treatment onset for polyarteritis nodosa, microscopic polyangiitis, and Churg-Strauss syndrome: a retrospective analysis of causes and factors predictive of mortality based on 595 patients. Medicine (Baltimore) 2005;84: 323–30.
60. Sable-Fourtassou R, Cohen P, Mahr A, et al. Antineutrophil cytoplasmic antibodies and the Churg-Strauss syndrome. Ann Intern Med 2005;143:632–8.
61. Keogh KA, Specks U. Churg-Strauss syndrome: clinical presentation, antineutrophil cytoplasmic antibodies, and leukotriene receptor antagonists. Am J Med 2003;115:284–90.
62. Churg J, Strauss L. Allergic granulomatosis, allergic angiitis, and periarteritis nodosa. Am J Pathol 1951;27:277–301.
63. Comarmond C, Pagnoux C, Khellaf M, et al. Eosinophilic granulomatosis with polyangiitis (Churg-Strauss): clinical characteristics and long-term followup of the 383 patients enrolled in the French Vasculitis Study Group cohort. Arthritis Rheum 2013;65:270–81.
64. Guillevin L, Cohen P, Gayraud M, et al. Churg-Strauss syndrome. Clinical study and long-term follow-up of 96 patients. Medicine (Baltimore) 1999;78:26–37.
65. Neumann T, Manger B, Schmid M, et al. Cardiac involvement in Churg-Strauss syndrome: impact of endomyocarditis. Medicine (Baltimore) 2009;88:236–43.
66. Dennert RM, van Paassen P, Schalla S, et al. Cardiac involvement in Churg-Strauss syndrome. Arthritis Rheum 2010;62:627–34.
67. Moosig F, Bremer JP, Hellmich B, et al. A vasculitis centre based management strategy leads to improved outcome in eosinophilic granulomatosis and polyangiitis (Churg-Strauss, EGPA): monocentric experiences in 150 patients. Ann Rheum Dis 2013;72:1011–7.

68. Sinico RA, Di Toma L, Maggiore U, et al. Prevalence and clinical significance of antineutrophil cytoplasmic antibodies in Churg-Strauss syndrome. Arthritis Rheum 2005;52:2926–35.
69. Baldini C, Talarico R, Della Rossa A, et al. Clinical manifestations and treatment of Churg-Strauss syndrome. Rheum Dis Clin North Am 2010;36:527–43.
70. Vinit J, Bielefeld P, Muller G, et al. Heart involvement in Churg-Strauss syndrome: retrospective study in French Burgundy population in past 10 years. Eur J Intern Med 2010;21:341–6.
71. Leon-Ruiz L, Jimenez-Alonso J, Hidalgo-Tenorio C, et al. Churg-Strauss syndrome complicated by endomyocardial fibrosis and intraventricular thrombus. Importance of the echocardiography for the diagnosis of asymptomatic phases of potentially severe cardiac complications. Lupus 2002;11:765–7.
72. Kajihara H, Kato Y, Takanashi A, et al. Periarteritis of coronary arteries with severe eosinophilic infiltration. A new pathologic entity (eosinophilic periarteritis)? Pathol Res Pract 1988;184:46–52.
73. Taira K, Tsunoda R, Watanabe T, et al. An autopsy case of isolated eosinophilic coronary periarteritis: a limited form of Churg-Strauss syndrome or a new entity? Intern Med 2005;44:586–9.
74. Lepper PM, Koenig W, Moller P, et al. A case of sudden cardiac death due to isolated eosinophilic coronary arteritis. Chest 2005;128:1047–50.
75. Stoukas V, Dragovic LJ. Sudden deaths from eosinophilic coronary monoarteritis: a subset of spontaneous coronary artery dissection. Am J Forensic Med Pathol 2009;30:268–9.
76. Mahrholdt H, Goedecke C, Wagner A, et al. Cardiovascular magnetic resonance assessment of human myocarditis: a comparison to histology and molecular pathology. Circulation 2004;109:1250–8.
77. Bohl S, Wassmuth R, Abdel-Aty H, et al. Delayed enhancement cardiac magnetic resonance imaging reveals typical patterns of myocardial injury in patients with various forms of non-ischemic heart disease. Int J Cardiovasc Imaging 2008;24:597–607.
78. Morita H, Yokoyama I, Yamada N, et al. Usefulness of 18FDG/13N-ammonia PET imaging for evaluation of the cardiac damage in Churg-Strauss syndrome. Eur J Nucl Med Mol Imaging 2004;31:1218.
79. Marmursztejn J, Guillevin L, Trebossen R, et al. Churg-Strauss syndrome cardiac involvement evaluated by cardiac magnetic resonance imaging and positron-emission tomography: a prospective study on 20 patients. Rheumatology (Oxford) 2013;52(4):642–50.
80. Vaglio A, Moosig F, Zwerina J. Churg-Strauss syndrome: update on pathophysiology and treatment. Curr Opin Rheumatol 2012;24:24–30.
81. Hellmich B, Csernok E, Gross WL. Proinflammatory cytokines and autoimmunity in Churg-Strauss syndrome. Ann N Y Acad Sci 2005;1051:121–31.
82. Peen E, Hahn P, Lauwers G, et al. Churg-Strauss syndrome: localization of eosinophil major basic protein in damaged tissues. Arthritis Rheum 2000;43:1897–900.
83. Cohen P, Pagnoux C, Mahr A, et al. Churg-Strauss syndrome with poor-prognosis factors: a prospective multicenter trial comparing glucocorticoids and six or twelve cyclophosphamide pulses in forty-eight patients. Arthritis Rheum 2007;57:686–93.
84. Ribi C, Cohen P, Pagnoux C, et al. Treatment of Churg-Strauss syndrome without poor-prognosis factors: a multicenter, prospective, randomized, open-label study of seventy-two patients. Arthritis Rheum 2008;58:586–94.

85. Forstot JZ, Overlie PA, Neufeld GK, et al. Cardiac complications of Wegener granulomatosis: a case report of complete heart block and review of the literature. Semin Arthritis Rheum 1980;10:148–54.

86. Eisen A, Arnson Y, Dovrish Z, et al. Arrhythmias and conduction defects in rheumatological diseases–a comprehensive review. Semin Arthritis Rheum 2009;39: 145–56.

87. Hoffman GS, Kerr GS, Leavitt RY, et al. Wegener granulomatosis: an analysis of 158 patients. Ann Intern Med 1992;116:488–98.

88. Wegener's Granulomatosis Etanercept Trial (WGET) Research Group. Etanercept plus standard therapy for Wegener's granulomatosis. N Engl J Med 2005;352:351–61.

89. Stone JH, Merkel PA, Spiera R, et al. Rituximab versus cyclophosphamide for ANCA-associated vasculitis. N Engl J Med 2010;363:221–32.

90. Lacoste C, Mansencal N, Ben M'rad M, et al. Valvular involvement in ANCA-associated systemic vasculitis: a case report and literature review. BMC Musculoskelet Disord 2011;12:50.

91. Herbst A, Padilla MT, Prasad AR, et al. Cardiac Wegener's granulomatosis masquerading as left atrial myxoma. Ann Thorac Surg 2003;75:1321–3.

92. Walton EW. Giant-cell granuloma of the respiratory tract (Wegener's granulomatosis). Br Med J 1958;2:265–70.

93. Oliveira GH, Seward JB, Tsang TS, et al. Echocardiographic findings in patients with Wegener granulomatosis. Mayo Clin Proc 2005;80:1435–40.

94. Guillevin L, Durand-Gasselin B, Cevallos R, et al. Microscopic polyangiitis: clinical and laboratory findings in eighty-five patients. Arthritis Rheum 1999;42:421–30.

95. Terrier B, Karras A, Cluzel P, et al. Presentation and prognosis of cardiac involvement in hepatitis C virus-related vasculitis. Am J Cardiol 2013;111: 265–72.

96. Rieu V, Cohen P, Andre MH, et al. Characteristics and outcome of 49 patients with symptomatic cryoglobulinaemia. Rheumatology (Oxford) 2002;41:290–300.

97. Gorevic PD, Kassab HJ, Levo Y, et al. Mixed cryoglobulinemia: clinical aspects and long-term follow-up of 40 patients. Am J Med 1980;69:287–308.

98. Zaidan M, Mariotte E, Galicier L, et al. Vasculitic emergencies in the intensive care unit: a special focus on cryoglobulinemic vasculitis. Ann Intensive Care 2012;2:31.

99. Geri G, Wechsler B, Thi Huong du L, et al. Spectrum of cardiac lesions in Behcet disease: a series of 52 patients and review of the literature. Medicine (Baltimore) 2012;91:25–34.

100. Zhu YL, Wu QJ, Guo LL, et al. The clinical characteristics and outcome of intracardiac thrombus and aortic valvular involvement in Behcet's disease: an analysis of 20 cases. Clin Exp Rheumatol 2012;30:S40–5.

101. Kaneko Y, Tanaka K, Yoshizawa A, et al. Successful treatment of recurrent intracardiac thrombus in Behcet's disease with immunosuppressive therapy. Clin Exp Rheumatol 2005;23:885–7.

Cardiovascular Disease in Rheumatoid Arthritis

Deepali Sen, MBBS*, María González-Mayda, MD,
Richard D. Brasington Jr, MD

KEYWORDS

- Rheumatoid arthritis • Cardiovascular disease • Inflammation • Atherosclerosis
- Management

KEY POINTS

- Rheumatoid arthritis (RA) is associated with significant cardiovascular disease burden.
- Atherosclerotic cardiovascular disease is a major cause of mortality in RA.
- Uncontrolled inflammation in RA predisposes to atherosclerosis.
- Tight disease control is key to reducing cardiovascular disease in RA.

INTRODUCTION

Rheumatoid arthritis (RA) is the most common inflammatory arthritis. As more effective therapies for RA became available, it was identified that patients with RA still had higher mortality compared with the general population. Cardiac disease was recognized as a major cause of morbidity and mortality in RA and became a topic of intense focus and research over the past decade. Much progress has been made into understanding the epidemiology of cardiac disease in RA from large cohorts of patients. The link between inflammation in RA and accelerated atherosclerosis has also become apparent. The burden of subclinical cardiac disease and cardiovascular disease (CVD) as a cause of death was apparent even in early autopsy series.[1] In a recently published autopsy series of 369 patients with RA from 1952 to 1991 the investigators reported that 221 (60%) patients had some form of CVD. In this cohort from the pre-biological era, the investigators reported significantly more incidence of cardiac amyloidosis and myopericarditis than the control population.[2] Outside atherosclerotic disease, cardiac involvement as an extra-articular manifestation of RA itself is also fairly prevalent. Newer imaging techniques and diagnostic modalities like

Funding Support: None.
Disclosure: Dr Brasington: Speaker for Pfizer, Clinical trials for Actelion and Savient.
Division of Rheumatology, Department of Medicine, Campus Box 8045, Washington University School of Medicine, 660 South Euclid Avenue, St Louis, MO 63110, USA
* Corresponding author.
E-mail address: dsen@dom.wustl.edu

echocardiograms and cardiac magnetic resonance imaging (MRI) have also shown that subclinical cardiac disease is highly prevalent in RA. In this article, both atherosclerotic and nonatherosclerotic cardiac manifestations in RA are reviewed.

CARDIAC DISEASE AS AN EXTRA-ARTICULAR MANIFESTATION OF RA
Pericarditis

Pericarditis is believed to be the most common cardiac manifestation of RA. Although clinically symptomatic pericarditis in RA occurs in less than 5% of patients, evidence of pericardial involvement is seen in 20% to 50% of patients by echocardiography.[3–5] Autopsy series similarly report that 20% to 40% of patients have evidence of pericarditis, which is mostly fibrinous.[2,3]

Pericarditis is frequently seen in male patients, in those who are seropositive, and in patients who have severe or active disease. Pericarditis can be either constrictive or effusive. Pericardial fluid tends to have a high protein count and lactate dehydrogenase level and however, it has a low glucose level. Cholesterol crystals may also be found.[6] Clinically symptomatic patients may present with chest pain or dyspnea. A pericardial rub may be present. Hemodynamic compromise caused by pericardial disease is infrequent and is seen in about 0.5% of patients.[7] Pericarditis does not always parallel joint inflammation. In rare instances, patients may have pericarditis in the setting of positive serologies for RA in the absence of significant joint symptoms. Echocardiography, chest computed tomography (CT), or a right heart catheterization may be necessary to make a diagnosis of pericardial involvement, especially if there is constrictive disease. CT may show pericardial inflammation, fluid, or calcification.

Treatment can include nonsteroidal antiinflammatory drugs (NSAIDs), steroids, disease-modifying antirheumatic drugs (DMARDs), or biological DMARDS therapy. There is evidence to suggest that biological therapy reduces occurrence of extra-articular manifestations of RA.[8] On the other hand, there are case reports of pericarditis developing in patients receiving biological therapy, and in this situation, infection and malignancy need to be ruled out.[9] Patients who have hemodynamic compromise should undergo surgical intervention like pericardiectomy or pericardial window. In 1 series,[7] patients with RA who developed hemodynamic compromise as a result of pericardial involvement had 100% mortality at 2 years. Thus, surgical intervention should not be deferred for a trial of medical therapy because fluid can reaccumulate on medical therapy alone and lead to serious consequences.

Valvular Heart Disease

Although valvular disease has not been considered to be a major cardiac manifestation of RA, echocardiographic studies have revealed a higher than anticipated incidence of asymptomatic valvular involvement. Mitral valve involvement is the most common, with echocardiographic evidence of valve thickening extending into the valve ring and subvalvular apparatus. Histologically, valves may show fibrosis or nodules.[3] Disease may at times be severe, leading to valvulitis, regurgitation, or rupture. Transthoracic echocardiographic (TTE) studies have estimated the incidence of asymptomatic valvular abnormalities from 24% to 39%.[5,10,11]

Two studies using transesophageal echocardiography (TEE) as the imaging modality show an even higher incidence of asymptomatic valvular disease. When Guedes and colleagues[12] performed TTE on 30 unselected patients with RA without known cardiac disease, only 2 patients had normal studies, and 25 of 30 (83%) had evidence of valvular disease compared with 53% of controls. Mitral regurgitation was seen in 24 of 30 (80%) of patients. Nodular involvement of valves was identified in 2 patients, and

11 of 30 (37%) had evidence of cardiomyopathy. Another study by Roldan and colleagues[13] looked at TEE findings in 34 patients with RA; 20 of 34 (59%) had evidence of left-sided valvular involvement, 11 of 34 (32%) had valve nodules. One patient had evidence of Libman-Sacks endocarditis. A meta-analysis looking at 10 echocardiographic studies of patients with RA with asymptomatic cardiac involvement reported 4 times the incidence of valvular thickening and calcification, and 5 times the incidence of valve nodules in patients with RA compared with controls.[14] One study[15] noted higher valvular involvement in patients with nodular versus nonnodular RA. Calcific deposits on valves have also been noted and are believed to be reflective of coronary atherosclerotic disease.[16]

Myocardial Disease

Congestive heart failure (CHF) is a major cause of morbidity and mortality in RA, accounting for about 20% of mortality in patients with RA.[17] Although several risk factors for myocardial disease like diabetes mellitus (DM), hypertension (HTN), and dyslipidemia are increased in RA, studies suggest that the risk of CHF in RA is higher than accounted for by these traditional risk factors. The CHF risk is high in patients with RA even after adjustment for underlying ischemic heart disease.[18] In a study by Nicola and colleagues,[19] among a cohort of 575 patients with RA and 583 controls who were followed for 30 years, the incidence of CHF was 34% in patients with RA versus 25.2% in patients who did not have RA ($P<.001$). RA increased the risk of CHF even after adjusting for demographics, ischemic heart disease, and other risk factors. In a study of 795 patients with RA followed for an average of 9.7 years, 92 developed CHF. Erythrocyte sedimentation rate (ESR), rheumatoid factor (RF) positivity, extra-articular involvement, and steroid use were the factors that remained associated with risk of CHF after adjusting for coronary artery disease and other traditional cardiovascular risk factors.[20] This finding suggests that RA is an independent risk factor for CHF.

Recently, myocardial involvement, especially in the form of diastolic dysfunction (DD), has been reported in RA. Several large studies using TTE have documented higher rates of DD in RA compared with controls.[11,21–26] DD is reported in up to 66% of patients with RA in some studies, and most patients tend to be clinically asymptomatic. There are no conclusive data linking DD to either the duration or the severity of RA.[27]

In a recent meta-analysis of 25 studies that included 1614 matched patients with RA, the most frequently reported echocardiographic abnormality was a prolonged isovolumetric relaxation time or a lower E/A ratio, which signify impaired ventricular relaxation. Most studies reported preserved ejection fraction and some evidence of right heart involvement with either right ventricular DD or increased pulmonary pressures.[28]

Myocardial involvement is found in up to 30% of cases in autopsy series, and most cases remain clinically asymptomatic. Histologically, the myocardial disease can be diffuse or focal; there may be myocardial granulomas or necrosis. Sometimes, fibrosis can be found as well.[3]

The incidence of progression to clinically significant CHF is low. Correa de Sa and colleagues[29] reported that in patients with evidence of DD the probability of developing CHF at 2 years is 1.9%, and the probability of developing cardiac related symptoms at 2 years was 31.1%. A study that looked at the 5-year follow-up of patients suggests that the rate of progression of DD may be independent of the RA disease activity, and similar to progression in patients who do not have RA.[25]

DD in the general population is associated with increased left ventricular mass. In RA, there are conflicting results regarding the associations of left ventricular mass to DD. In a meta-analysis, Corrao and colleagues[30] analyzed the data from

4 echocardiographic studies and concluded that patients with RA tended to have an increase in left ventricular mass. This finding is by contrast to cardiac MRI in the study by Giles and colleagues,[31] who reported that patients with RA tended to have lower left ventricular volumes, with an average of 26 g or 18% lower in patients with RA compared with age-matched controls ($P<.001$). The ventricular volumes were inversely associated with anti-cyclic citrullinated peptide (anti-CCP) antibody titers and with biological use. Myocardial dysfunction is believed to be caused by microvascular changes that occur because of inflammatory cytokines like tumor necrosis factor α (TNF-α), interleukin 1 (IL-1), and IL-6, which lead to myocardial remodeling and fibrosis. A study by Davis and colleagues[32] evaluated 212 patients with RA for presence and severity of DD by TTE and measured the release of 17 cytokines by blood mononuclear cells in response to stimulation. These investigators noted that an 11-cytokine profile was able to distinguish patients with moderate to severe DD compared with patients with normal heart function. More recently, myocardial tissue from patients with RA was found to have higher levels of citrullination of proteins compared with controls, which may account for myocardial involvement in RA.[33]

Myocardial Dysfunction Related to RA Medication

Another aspect of myocardial dysfunction in RA is medication toxicity, especially TNF inhibitors (TNF-I) and antimalarial agents. Antimalarial medication hydroxychloroquine (HCQ) is commonly used in RA. Most of the cardiotoxicity associated with antimalarial medications has generally involved chloroquine,[34] although there are several case reports of cardiotoxicity with HCQ.[35–42] Although most case reports are related to long-term use of HCQ, there are reports of cardiotoxicity occurring early and with variable cumulative doses.[34,43] The defect might be restrictive, there may be enlargement of ventricles or atria, and biventricular failure may result. Diagnosis cannot be made with certainty in the absence of histopathology, which typically shows vacuolar changes. Myelin figures and curvilinear bodies that represent abnormal lysosomes are also specific to antimalarial cardiotoxicity. Biopsy may also be necessary to rule out other diagnoses like myocarditis and amyloidosis. Similar histologic changes are observed with antimalarial-associated neuromyopathy. Skeletal muscle involvement often coexists with cardiac involvement. In the literature review by Costedoat-Chalumeau and colleagues,[34] antimalarial-associated cardiotoxicity had high mortality (11/25 patients). Withdrawal of the medication resulted in stabilization in some cases (8/12 patients). There are case reports of patients who have required heart transplantation after antimalarial cardiotoxicity.[44]

Cardiomyopathy has also occurred with TNF-I. Although symptomatic heart failure is a contraindication to use of TNF- I, the risk of heart failure associated with anti-TNF agents is a controversial topic. Attention to possible worsening effects of TNF-I on CHF were brought into focus by 2 randomized controlled trials of TNF-I therapy in heart failure. More than a decade ago, high levels of TNF were found to be associated with heart failure.[45] Animal model studies also suggested that TNF may be involved in remodeling of the heart and that TNF inhibition may be beneficial in heart failure.[46,47] Inflammatory cytokines were believed to increase risk of CHF. This theory coupled with a successful phase 1 study of etanercept in heart failure[48] led to large randomized controlled trials of TNF-I agents in advanced symptomatic heart failure. Two studies were performed using etanercept, the North American RENNAISSANCE (Randomized Etanercept North American Strategy to Study Antagonism of Cytokines) and the European RECOVER (Research into Etanercept Cytokine Antagonism in Ventricular Dysfunction) trials, which together had a total of 2048 patients.[49] The ATTACH (Anti TNF-alpha Therapy Against Chronic Heart Failure) trial looked at the efficacy of infliximab in CHF.[50] All studies showed unfavorable outcomes, and both RENNAIS-SANCE and RECOVER were terminated prematurely because of worse outcomes in the treatment group. The ATTACH trial was also associated with adverse outcomes and clinical worsening, including mortality. The US Food and Drug Administration has since issued a warning against use of TNF-I in symptomatic CHF. Subsequently, about 47 cases of new or worsening cases of CHF have been noted in 300,000 patients treated with TNF-I worldwide.[51]

However, there are contrasting results from observational cohorts and various RA registries that do not show an increased risk of CHF in patients with RA treated with TNF-I. These studies report data for many patients from registries around the world, including the American registry,[18] Swedish registry,[52] British registry,[53] Spanish regis-try,[54] German registry,[55] and from the Veterans Administration.[56] All studies suggest that patients with RA who are treated with TNF-I have an overall lower or comparable prevalence of CHF compared with patients not treated with TNF-I. A recent meta-analysis of data from these registries[57] also concluded that patients with RA treated with TNF-I had a lower incidence of CHF than patients who did not receive this agent.

Because there is an intrinsic higher risk of CHF in RA, it is unclear if the unexplained cases of CHF were truly related to TNF-I.[55] Beneficial cardiac effects with TNF-I seen in the registries are retrospective observational data. This benefit also may be reflec-tive of the overall better control of inflammation, rather than effects specific to a class of drugs. Similar benefits are also seen with methotrexate.

Cardiac Amyloidosis

Reactive amyloid A deposition occurs in RA as a result of long-term, uncontrolled inflammation. An autopsy series of 161 patients with RA from 1970 to 1989 described amyloid deposition in 21% of patients with RA.[58] Another larger series of 369 au-topsies from 1952 to 1991 showed amyloidosis in 30% of patients with RA, with car-diac involvement in 28%.[59]

Although older studies tend to have higher incidence of amyloidosis, it is unknown what the incidence is in the biological DMARD era. Also, the higher incidence on au-topsy series may not be clinically relevant, because premortem diagnosis is rare. Studies looking at abdominal fat pad aspirates for diagnosis[60,61] estimate the inci-dence of systemic amyloidosis to be between 7% and 78% in patients with RA. Car-diac amyloidosis causes biventricular enlargement with DD. A characteristic sparkling pattern in the myocardium is evident on cardiac MRI. Evidence of renal or other organ involvement may be apparent in most patients. The incidence of amyloidosis is likely related to the severity and duration of inflammation. There is evidence that biological therapy, especially with anti-TNF agents, can reverse amyloid deposition.[62,63]

Coronary Arteritis

Early autopsy series[64,65] report up to 20% incidence of coronary vasculitis; these were reported before the advent of DMARD therapy. Coronary arteritis may result in cardiac ischemia or CHF. Because both ischemic heart disease and CHF are commonly seen in RA, it may be important to keep vasculitis as a differential diagnosis. An endomyo-cardial biopsy may be needed to differentiate cardiac ischemia caused by vasculitis from a similar picture caused by atherosclerotic disease.[66]

ATHEROSCLEROTIC DISEASE IN RA

Accelerated coronary artery and cerebrovascular atherosclerosis is a major cause of morbidity and mortality in RA. A meta-analysis by Avina-Zubieta and colleagues,[67] which included 14 studies and comprised 41,490 patients with RA, showed a 48% increased risk of cardiovascular events (CVD) compared with the general population. Patients with RA in these multiple studies were also noted to have a 68%, 41%, and 87% increase risk of myocardial infarction (MI), cerebrovascular accident (CVA), and CHF, respectively. Patients with RA are also prone to recurrent cardiac events,[68] and a higher mortality is noted in patients with RA after acute cardiovascular events.[69]

Both traditional risk factors, such as DM, dyslipidemia, obesity, HTN, and smoking, along with nontraditional risk factors, such as RA disease duration, seropositivity, and disease activity, play a role in increasing the risk of CVD in these patients. There are similarities between the inflammation occurring in the synovium and the inflammation occurring in the atherosclerotic plaque.[70] Proinflammatory cytokines that are present in the synovium and that clinically cause joint swelling, pain, warmth, and stiffness in patients with RA likely mediate similar effects on the cardiovascular system and other distant organs. Chronic inflammation can affect plaque formation and stability, vascular wall stiffness, and thrombogenic potential.

Traditional Risk Factors for CVD in RA

Dyslipidemia

In contrast to the general population, in whom increased lipid levels, particularly low-density lipoprotein (LDL), can increase the risk of cardiovascular events, it is decreased lipid levels that are associated with an increased cardiovascular risk in patients with RA. Inflammation in untreated RA as well as treatment of RA can affect lipid levels. Myasoedova and colleagues[71] performed a longitudinal population-based study that compared the lipid profiles of patients with RA with controls who did not have RA 5 years before and 5 years after the development of RA. These investigators found that there was a significant decline in LDL and total cholesterol levels in the RA group 5 years before they fulfilled American College of Rheumatology criteria, whereas there were no changes in the control group. Five years after diagnosis, patients with RA had LDL and total cholesterol levels similar to the control group. The investigators also noted a significant decrease in total cholesterol/high-density lipoprotein (HDL) ratio during the 5-year period before RA incidence.

This decrease in the total cholesterol, LDL, and HDL levels in patients with RA is believed to be caused by the presence of underlying inflammation. HDL levels are disproportionately decreased compared with the total cholesterol levels. This situation leads to an increase of total cholesterol/HDL ratio, which is also known as the atherogenic index. Myasoedova and colleagues[72] looked at 651 patients with RA and followed them for about 8 years. Lipid levels, inflammatory markers, cardiovascular risk factors, and the development of cardiovascular events were documented at each visit. An increased ESR was associated with significantly increased risk of CVD (particularly CHF) and mortality, adjusting for age, sex, and year of RA diagnosis. The higher the ESR/C-reactive protein (CRP) levels, the higher the risk of a CVD event and mortality, as would be expected. CRP was significantly associated with risk of CHF and mortality ($P = .07$). Increased levels of triglycerides were significantly associated with CVD. Lower total cholesterol and higher HDL levels were significantly associated with risk of CHF and persisted after adjustment for traditional cardiovascular risk factors. Lower LDL values were also associated with higher risk of MI.

There is evidence to suggest that HDL molecules in patients with RA are not only quantitatively low but also qualitatively abnormal. Proinflammatory HDL molecules are seen in RA, which do not prevent LDL oxidation.[73,74] Oxidized LDL particles are highly antigenic and cause antibody formation. Antioxidized LDL antibodies are also positively correlated with thickness of the carotid intima media.[75]

Other qualitative abnormalities include small dense LDL molecules, which are considered more atherogenic and are seen in greater proportion in patients with RA.[76] Lipoprotein A, which increases cardiovascular risk, was also found to be increased in patients with RA.[77]

Lipid profile is also affected by treatment of RA. Cholesterol, especially HDL levels, is known to increase in patients with RA after treatment. This finding is more pronounced in responders.[78,79] There is also a favorable shift in the total cholesterol/HDL ratio in treated RA. HCQ use is independently associated with lower LDL, total cholesterol, LDL/HDL, and total cholesterol/HDL ratio in patients with RA.[80]

Therapy with TNF-I increase total cholesterol and HDL levels without an equivalent effect on LDL levels. In a recent meta-analysis of 15 studies with a total of 766 patients,[81] anti-TNF therapy resulted in a 10% increase in total cholesterol and a 7% increase in HDL within the first 2 to 6 weeks of therapy.

The IL-6 receptor inhibitor tocilizumab causes increase in total cholesterol, LDL, and HDL as well as triglyceride levels.[82,83] Around 30% of patients treated with tocilizumab have increased lipid levels; this effect is dose dependent. In a study looking at cumulative data from 5 phase 3 trials, increase in LDL levels from less than 130 mg/dL at baseline to 130 mg/dL or higher with treatment were seen in 25.1% of patients treated with tocilizumab 4 mg/kg, 33.2% in patients treated with tocilizumab 8 mg/kg, and in 14.2% of controls. The increase in LDL levels occurred within the first 6 weeks of therapy.[84] The ACT-STAR study was a postapproval study designed to evaluate the safety of tocilizumab in a setting mimicking clinical practice. Of 886 patients with RA in this study, 11% had an increase in LDL levels that required initiation of statin therapy.[85] Combined data from clinical trials suggest that dyslipidemia caused by tocilizumab is not associated with an increased risk of cardiovascular events.[86] The Janus Kinus inhibitor tofacitinib increases both LDL and HDL levels.[87,88] Brumester and colleagues[89] reported that 10.9% of patients treated with tofacitinib 5 mg, 10% of patients treated with tofacitinib 10 mg, and 7% of controls had increases in LDL levels from a baseline of less than 100 mg/dL to greater than 130 mg/dL at 3 months of therapy.

The diverse effects of the different biological agents on lipids may be reflective of the role of individual cytokines on lipid metabolism.

Studies suggest that statin therapy in RA may alter lipid profile toward a favorable total cholesterol/LDL ratio, thereby decreasing cardiovascular risk. There is also evidence that statin therapy reduces inflammatory markers like CRP in RA.[90] Statin therapy in RA has efficacy in primary prevention of CVD as well as improving all-cause mortality.[91] Because of the immunomodulatory and antiinflammatory properties of statins, some studies have looked at the effects of statins on inflammation in RA. There is some evidence that statin therapy has modest antiinflammatory effects in RA. McCarey and colleagues[90] reported reduction in disease activity scores as well as inflammatory markers like CRP and ESR with atorvastatin use in RA. Another small study of 100 patients with RA[92] reported a statistically nonsignificant improvement in disease activity in patients receiving simvastatin 20 mg. Studies also report improvement in surrogate markers of CVD like arterial stiffness and flow-mediated dilatation in patients with RA treated with statins.[93–95] The TRACE-RA study has linked abrupt discontinuation of statins in RA to an increased risk of MI.[96]

HTN

HTN has been reported in 29% to 70% of patients with RA.[97] Overall prevalence of HTN is not believed to be higher in patients with RA compared with patients who do not have RA.[98] However, a few studies have reported a higher incidence of HTN in RA.[99,100] This discrepancy may be because HTN, especially in younger patients with RA, may remain undiagnosed. HTN is associated with RA medications like NSAIDs, glucocorticoids, and some DMARDs, like cyclosporine. HTN remains an independent risk factor for CVD in RA.

Insulin resistance

Contrary to anticipated risk, incidence of diabetes has not been found be increased in RA.[101,102] However, there is a strong association between RA and insulin resistance. Insulin resistance is found to be an independent risk factor of CVD in RA.[103] Insulin resistance was noted in 51% of early patients with RA and 58% of long-standing patients with RA compared with only 19% in controls, suggesting that inflammation plays a role in the development of insulin resistance.[104] Insulin resistance is believed to be mediated by inflammatory response in RA, especially mediated through TNF-α.[105] TNF-α has been shown to be expressed in both adipose tissue and muscle[106–108] and may play a role in insulin resistance by decreasing insulin-dependent glucose uptake by inhibiting autophosphorylation of the insulin receptor.[109]

TNF-α has also been implicated in insulin resistance in patients who do not have RA. Nilsson and colleagues[110] looked at 40, 70-year-old men with non–insulin-dependent DM (NIDDM) and compared them with 20 age-matched controls. Of the 40 men with NIDDM, 20 had severe insulin resistance, whereas the other 20 had moderate insulin resistance. The investigators measured serum TNF-α levels in all 3 groups. The serum TNF-α level in the control group was 3.27 ± 0.29 pg/mL, which was similar to levels in healthy men in previous studies. The serum TNF-α levels in the group with moderate resistance to insulin were 23% higher, whereas levels were 51% higher in the group with severe resistance to insulin ($P<.001$). These findings support TNF-α playing a role in insulin resistance and DM, especially in patients with RA, who have systemically increased levels of TNF-α. Therefore, patients with RA should be screened at least annually, especially if they have other risk factors for the development of DM, such as obesity, HTN, and dyslipidemia.

RA has been considered as an independent risk factor for the development of CVD similar to DM. Patients with type 2 DM and nondiabetic patients with RA were found to have similar hazard ratios (HRs) for CVD compared with the nondiabetic general population; HR of 2.04 (95% confidence interval [CI] 1.12–3.67, $P = .019$) versus 2.16 (95% CI 1.28–3.63, $P = .004$), respectively.[111]

Age

Crowson and colleagues[112] looked at a cohort of 563 patients with RA without a previous history of cardiovascular events and followed them on average for 8.2 years. In that period, 98 of the patients developed a cardiovascular event (74 of them were seropositive, whereas 24 were seronegative). However, the Framingham risk score for that same group predicted only 59.7 events. The investigators suggested that aging may have an accelerated effect on cardiovascular events in seropositive patients with RA, because the risk of cardiovascular events in seronegative patients with RA was similar to the general population.

Body mass index

Contrary to the general population, in RA a low body mass index (BMI, calculated as weight in kilograms divided by the square of height in meters) has been shown to be associated with an increase in cardiovascular events and mortality.[113] Chung and colleagues[104] used both the World Health Organization (WHO) and National Cholesterol Education Program (NCEP) Adult Treatment Panel III criteria to determine the prevalence of metabolic syndrome in 154 patients with RA. Eighty-eight of these patients had early RA defined as median disease lasting 2 years, whereas 66 of these patients had long-standing RA defined as median disease duration lasting 20 years. These patients were compared with 85 control individuals. Using the NCEP criteria, 30% of patients with early RA, 42% of patients with long-standing RA, and 22% of the controls had metabolic syndrome ($P = .03$). Using the WHO criteria, 31% of patients with early RA, 42% of patients with long-standing RA, and 11% of control patients met the definition of metabolic syndrome ($P<.001$). There was an increased prevalence of metabolic syndrome in individuals with RA whose BMI was 30 kg/m^2 or less. The statistical models performed in this study suggested that in RA, metabolic syndrome was independent of BMI, which goes against the classic definition of metabolic syndrome in the general population, in which obesity is a major component. These investigators also measured coronary artery calcification by electron beam CT, which is a reproducible and quantitative method for detection of coronary artery atherosclerosis, which can help in predicting future cardiovascular risk. After adjustment for age and sex, coronary artery calcification was statistically significantly associated with insulin resistance (odds ratio = 2.42, 95% CI: 1.22–4.79, $P = .01$) Weight loss in RA, termed rheumatoid cachexia, is mediated through TNF-α, and lower BMI in RA could indicate higher cytokine levels, which contributes to insulin resistance.

Smoking
The link between smoking and increased susceptibility to RA is well established.[114,115] Smoking is also associated with RA disease severity.[116] Past and active cigarette smoking have been associated with enhanced formation of IL-6.[117] Smoking is an independent risk factor for CVD in RA. Gerli and colleagues[118] found that among their cohort of 101 patients with RA, smoking status, number of smoking years, number of daily cigarettes, and cigarette years were all associated with increased thickness of the carotid mean intima media ($P<.05$ in all patients) when compared with nonsmokers.

Cardiovascular Risk Factors Associated with RA

Disease duration and its impact on CVD
Early RA has become an important concept in the treatment of RA, referring to a window of opportunity when effective treatment has the potential to change the disease course. Reports from several cohorts suggest that CVD risk is increased in early RA.[119,120] Goodson and colleagues[121] followed a total of 1236 patients with early RA over a median duration of 6.9 years. During this time, 160 patients died of a cardiovascular event; most were seropositive. Surrogate markers of vascular disease, like carotid intima media thickness, is also abnormal in patients with early RA compared with controls.[122,123] Although the onset of CVD is seen early, the risk continues to increase with disease duration. Cardiovascular mortality in established disease is known to increase in proportion to disease duration.[124,125]

Seropositivity and presence of shared epitope
It is known that RF-positive and CCP-positive patients tend to have more severe joint damage and extra-articular manifestations.[126] RF positivity has been associated with overall mortality.[127] Goodson and colleagues[121] reported that even in the earliest stages, patients with RF-positive inflammatory polyarthritis have a higher risk of death from CVD causes than do RF-negative patients. Gerli and colleagues[128] evaluated the effect of anti-CCP on atherosclerotic damage in RA, carotid intima media thickness of 81 consecutive patients with RA without overt CVD was analyzed by ultrasonography. Carotid intima media thickness values were higher in the patients with RA versus controls at all artery domains examined. Patients with RA with detectable circulating

anti-CCP had thicker carotid intima media at internal carotid arterial wall than patients without evidence of these antibodies.

The relationship of shared epitope with anti-CCP antibodies in RA is well known. Shared epitope alleles have also been associated with mortality in RA and with ischemic heart disease. In a study by Farragher and colleagues,[129] presence of 2 copies of shared epitope was associated with highest all-cause mortality. Combination of shared epitope, anti-CCP antibodies, and smoking predicted the highest risk of cardiovascular mortality in RA. Certain shared epitope genotypes, especially HLA-DRB1 0404, have been associated with increased risk in several studies.[130,131]

Inflammation as a risk factor for atherosclerosis

Baseline increased CRP levels have been linked to an increased risk of death from cardiovascular causes. This increased risk was also influenced by whether the patients were seropositive or negative for RF, because those with a baseline CRP level of 5 mg/L who were seronegative had a 1.5-fold increased risk of death from a cardiovascular cause versus a 7-fold increased risk of death from cardiovascular cause in RF-positive patients.[132] High CRP levels conferred risk of CVD even in patients whose disease was clinically quiescent.[133] High CRP levels were also found to correlate with thicker carotid intima media in a study involving 47 patients with RA.[134]

Inflammation has been shown to be involved in the pathogenesis of atherosclerosis. It leads to endothelial cell dysfunction, plaque rupture, and subsequent thrombosis.[135] Persistent inflammation stimulates arterial wall remodeling and foam cell formation, which are both a hallmark of early atherosclerotic lesion.[136] Similarities exist in the inflammatory response found in the rheumatoid synovium and atherosclerotic plaque. Cytokines like TNF-α and IL-6 are associated with pathogenesis of joint inflammation. These cytokines are also implicated in the increased cardiovascular risk seen in RA. IL-6 expression is seen in atherosclerotic plaques.[137] IL-6 is produced by vascular smooth muscle cells, and increased serums levels have been associated with intima media thickness and proliferation of the smooth muscle cells.[138] High IL-6 levels are also associated with high CRP levels, which is a known association of CVD. People with high levels of IL-6 are 2 to 5 times more likely to have a heart attack, stroke, or other cardiovascular episodes, as shown by the study of Cesari and colleagues[139] TNF-α has also been detected in the endothelium, smooth muscle cells, and macrophages associated with coronary atherosclerotic plaques.[140]

Role of medications in cardiovascular risk in RA

NSAIDs NSAIDs are commonly used to help treat arthritic symptoms, given their potent antiinflammatory mechanism of action. However, in patients with a history of a previous MI, NSAID use should be limited as much as possible because of its increased risk of a repeat cardiovascular event. Schjerning and colleagues[141] followed 83,675 patients with a previous history of a MI. Of these patients, 42.3% were prescribed NSAIDs at least once during follow-up. NSAID treatment was associated with a significantly increased risk of death at the beginning of the treatment, and the increased risk persisted throughout the course of treatment (HR 1.45, 95% CI 1.29–1.62; and HR 1.55, 95% CI 1.46–1.64 after 90 days). Naproxen was not associated with an increased risk of death or MI for the entire treatment duration; however, diclofenac was linked to the highest risk. In their meta-analysis, Trelle and colleagues[142] showed that NSAIDs were linked to 46% of all cardiovascular deaths in 312 accumulated events from 26 trials. All drugs, except for naproxen, showed evidence of an increased risk of cardiovascular death compared with placebo.

In those patients with RA already taking an aspirin for secondary cardiovascular prevention, concurrent NSAID may decrease the antiplatelet effect of the former.[143] These investigators showed that there was an increase in the rate of a recurrent acute MI in patients exposed to both aspirin and ibuprofen compared with those taking aspirin alone (HR 1.01, 95% CI 0.58–1.76). After 30 days, the HR was 1.13, with a 95% CI between 0.54 and 2.39, and after more than 60 days, the HR increased to 1.83, with a 95% CI between 0.76 and 4.42. It is hypothesized that ibuprofen blocks the binding channel, so that aspirin is unable to bind to cyclooxygenase. Use of naproxen and aspirin for a period of 60 days or more led to a decrease in the rate of a recurrent acute MI when compared with those patients who took only aspirin.[143]

In contrast to the preceding discussion, 1 inception cohort from the Norfolk arthritis registry did not show any increase in cardiovascular risk in patients with RA treated with NSAIDs.[144] Lindhardsen and colleagues[145] showed that the cardiovascular risk in patients with RA taking NSAIDs was modest. These investigators conducted a longitudinal cohort study of 17,320 patients with RA followed on average for 5 years. A total of 6283 cardiovascular events occurred during that time. Cox regression stratified by RA status showed that overall, NSAID exposure was associated with a 22% risk increase in patients with RA compared with a 51% increase in patients who did not have RA. Rofecoxib (which was removed from the market in 2004) was associated with the highest risk in both patients with RA (HR 1.57) and controls (HR 2.19).

Glucocorticoids Steroids are associated with an increase in traditional cardiovascular risk factors. Cardiovascular risk with steroid use is dose dependent.[146]

This finding was shown by the study by Greenberg and colleagues,[147] in which prednisone dosages between 1 and 7 mg daily had an HR of 1.78 (95% CI 1.06–2.96) versus an HR of 2.62 (95% CI 1.29–2.96) for dosages of prednisone of 7.5 mg/d or greater. Davis and colleagues[148] retrospectively reviewed 603 patients with RA for their use of corticosteroids. Risk of cardiovascular events was assessed over 13 years. These investigators noted that those patients who were RF negative who had been exposed to glucocorticoids did not have an increased risk of cardiovascular events regardless of dosage or amount of use (HR 0.85, 95% CI 0.39–1.87), whereas RF-positive patients with a high cumulative exposure to corticosteroids had a 3-fold increased risk of cardiovascular events (HR 3.06, 95% CI 1.81–5.18).

In a study of 8384 patients with RA on corticosteroids, 298 cases of MIs were reported. Multivariable models showed that current use of corticosteroids was associated with a 68% increased risk of an MI. Separate multivariable models showed that current daily dose, cumulative duration of use, and total cumulative dose were all associated with a significant increased risk of MI.[149] These same investigators showed that glucocorticoids were not associated with an increased risk of strokes (CVA) in patients with RA, as shown by the population-based cohort of 7051 patients with RA followed over a median of 6 years. A total of 178 incident CVA cases were reported; however, this was not considered a significant increased risk of CVA (HR 1.41, 95% CI 0.84–2.37). Models that accounted for daily dose, cumulative duration of use, and total cumulative dose were also not significantly associated with CVA.[150]

Risk Assessment for CVD in RA

Assessing the risk of a cardiovascular event in patients with RA cannot be measured with the same tools used to measure cardiovascular risk in the general population. For example, using the Framingham risk score in patients with RA can underestimate the risk of developing a cardiovascular event, as shown by Crowson and colleagues,[151] who conducted a study comparing the observed and predicted cardiovascular risk in patients with RA versus controls using both the Framingham and the Reynolds risk score. The observed cardiovascular risk was significantly higher than the predicted risk in seropositive patients with RA, those with persistently increased ESRs, and in those older than 75 years. Using the Framingham risk score and the Reynolds risk score also underestimated the cardiovascular risk in women with RA with increased CRP levels. Overall, the Framingham risk score underestimated cardiovascular risk by 102% in women and 65% in men with RA.

This finding led to the European League Against Rheumatism (EULAR) proposing a risk score model, in which a multiplication factor of 1.5 is added to the risk score if a patient with RA meets 2 of the following 3 criteria: (1) disease duration of more than 10 years, (2) positive for RF or anti-CCP antibodies, or (3) the presence of certain extra-articular manifestations.[152]

The EULAR risk model has not been validated in large cohorts. The EULAR task force in its report mentioned that this correction of 1.5 is conservative. It is likely that the cardiovascular risk associated with RA may still be underestimated even after applying the numeric correction.[153] This theory may be especially true of patients with severe inflammation but disease duration of less than 10 years.[119,120] Applying the correction likely identifies additional patients in whom aggressive risk management and primary prevention can be implemented.

Management of Cardiovascular Risks in Patients with RA

In 2010, EULAR presented guidelines for management of cardiovascular risk in RA. They recommend that RA be considered as an independent risk factor for CVD. Adequate disease control is necessary for reducing cardiovascular risk. All patients with RA, especially those with active disease, should receive an annual CVD risk assessment, and if they have inactive disease, they may undergo CVD risk assessment every 2 to 3 years. Risk assessment should be adjusted for RA, and total cholesterol/HDL ratios should be used for assessing risk. Primary prevention strategies similar to those used in the general population should be used in patients with RA.[152]

Blood pressure, weight, physical activity, smoking status, and comorbidities, such as dyslipidemia and DM, should be monitored and discussed at each clinic visit. Fasting lipid panels should be checked on a regular basis, and treatment with statins should be implemented, if necessary. Statin therapy is useful for management of dyslipidemia as well as modulation of inflammatory response associated with atherosclerosis, as shown by decreasing of CRP levels. Some studies suggest that with adequate risk stratification, up to 22% of patients with RA without known CVD may meet indication for statin therapy. However, most of these patients are not treated adequately with statins.[154] Angiotensin-converting enzyme inhibitors and angiotensin receptor blockers should be used for HTN, because of their effects on the vasculature and endothelial stability in patients with RA.[155–157] NSAID use should be judicious in patients with known CVD. As discussed earlier, high doses of steroids have been associated with an increased risk of cardiovascular events in patients with RA. It is therefore recommended that if steroids are deemed necessary as part of the management, low doses should be used for the shortest period. Treatment should also include a multidisciplinary approach to ensure that all comorbidities are being addressed and appropriately controlled. Smoking cessation should be strongly advised at each visit, and the emphasis on its detrimental cardiovascular outcomes if patients continue to smoke should be discussed.

Cardiovascular Risk Reduction by Disease Control

Effective treatment of RA is associated with reduction in cardiovascular risk. Although both DMARD and biological DMARD therapy have been associated with benefit, some studies suggest that the benefit may be larger in patients treated with biologics, especially TNF-I therapy.[147]

However, several studies have documented cardiovascular risk reduction with methotrexate. Choi and colleagues[158] conducted a prospective study of 1240 patients with RA followed for an average of 6 years while being treated with various oral DMARDs including methotrexate, sulfasalazine, HCQ, penicillamine, and intramuscular gold. These investigators noted that cardiovascular deaths were decreased by 70% in patients treated with methotrexate. Several meta-analyses looking at data from large cohorts have also confirmed the lowering of cardiovascular risk with methotrexate.[159,160] El-Barbary and colleagues[161] showed that IL-6 and TNF-α are both increased in early active RA and these levels decrease and sometimes normalize with methotrexate therapy.

However, Greenberg and colleagues[147] found that treatment with TNF-I but not methotrexate was associated with a reduced risk of cardiovascular events when compared with nonbiological DMARDs. This risk reduction was observed for both MI and CVA as individual outcomes. TNF-I are known to have favorable effects on insulin resistance and lipid profiles in RA, which may explain this finding. In a recent study, the HR for cardiovascular events was 20% to 29% lower in patients receiving TNF-I compared with DMARD therapy; however, this benefit was seen for only up to 12 months of therapy.[162] This effect may be attributable to better and earlier disease control with biological agents rather than a class effect of biologics themselves.[163,164] TNF-I have also been shown to have beneficial effects on vascular stiffness, as measured by surrogate markers like aortic pulse wave velocity.[165–167] In the meta-analysis by Barnabe and colleagues,[168] TNF-I therapy was associated with greater risk reduction than DMARD therapy in observational cohorts but not randomized controlled studies.

SUMMARY

RA can manifest in a variety of cardiac complications, including pericarditis, valvular disease, cardiomyopathy, and amyloidosis. Subclinical involvement is higher than anticipated. CVD is also prevalent in patients with RA, with onset in early disease. Several disease-specific risk factors, like seropositivity, disease activity, and medications, are implicated in the pathogenesis of CVD in RA. Cardiovascular risk assessment in RA varies from the general population. Some traditional risk factors like BMI and lipid levels apply differently to the RA population. Statins are useful in managing dyslipidemia in RA. There is good evidence to support cardiovascular risk reduction with methotrexate and TNF-I use if good disease control is achieved.

REFERENCES

1. Mutru O, Koota K, Isomäki H. Causes of death in autopsied RA patients. Scand J Rheumatol 1976;5:239–40.
2. Koivuniemi R, Paimela L, Suomalainen R, et al. Cardiovascular diseases in patients with rheumatoid arthritis. Scand J Rheumatol 2013;42(2):131–5.
3. Kitas G, Banks M, Bacon P. Cardiac involvement in rheumatoid arthritis. Clin Med 2001;1:18–21.
4. Corrao A, Salli L, Arnone R, et al. Cardiac involvement in rheumatoid arthritis: evidence of silent heart disease. Eur Heart J 1995;16:253–6.

5. Mody GM, Stevens JE, Meyers OL. The heart in rheumatoid arthritis: a clinical and echocardiographic study. Q J Med 1987;65:921–8.

6. Barcin C, Yalcinkaya E, Kabul HK. Cholesterol pericarditis associated with rheumatoid arthritis: a rare cause of pericardial effusion. Int J Cardiol 2013;166(3): e56–8.

7. Escalante A, Kaufman RL, Quismorio FP Jr, et al. Cardiac compression in rheumatoid pericarditis. Semin Arthritis Rheum 1990;20(3):148–63.

8. Nyhäll-Wåhlin BM, Petersson IF, Jacobsson C, et al. Extra-articular manifestations in a community-based sample of patients with rheumatoid arthritis: incidence and relationship to treatment with TNF inhibitors. Scand J Rheumatol 2012;41:434–7.

9. Ambrose NL, O'Connell PG. Anti-TNF alpha therapy does not always protect rheumatoid arthritis patients against developing pericarditis. Clin Exp Rheumatol 2007;25(4):660.

10. Nagyhegyi G, Nades I, Banyai F, et al. Cardiac and cardiopulmonary disorders in patients with ankylosing spondylitis and rheumatoid arthritis. Clin Exp Rheumatol 1988;6:17–26.

11. Wisłowska M, Sypuła S, Kowalik I. Echocardiographic findings, 24-hour electrocardiographic Holter monitoring in patients with rheumatoid arthritis according to Steinbrocker's criteria, functional index, value of Waaler-Rose titre and duration of disease. Clin Rheumatol 1998;17(5):369–77.

12. Guedes C, Bianchi-Fior P, Cormier B, et al. Cardiac manifestations of rheumatoid arthritis: a case control transesophageal echocardiography study in 30 patients. Arthritis Care Res 2001;45:129–35.

13. Roldan CA, DeLong C, Qualls CR, et al. Characterization of valvular heart disease in rheumatoid arthritis by transesophageal echocardiography and clinical correlates. Am J Cardiol 2007;100(3):496–502.

14. Corrao S, Messina S, Pistone G, et al. Heart involvement in rheumatoid arthritis: systematic review and meta-analysis. Int J Cardiol 2013;167(5):2031–8.

15. Wisłowska M, Sypuła S, Kowalik I. Echocardiographic findings and 24-h electrocardiographic Holter monitoring in patients with nodular and non-nodular rheumatoid arthritis. Rheumatol Int 1999;18(5–6):163–9.

16. Yiu KH, Wang S, Mok MY, et al. Relationship between cardiac valvular and arterial calcification in patients with rheumatoid arthritis and systemic lupus erythematosus. J Rheumatol 2011;38(4):621–7.

17. Nicola PJ, Crowson CS, Maradit-Kremers H, et al. Contribution of congestive heart failure and ischemic heart disease to excess mortality in rheumatoid arthritis. Arthritis Rheum 2006;54:60–7.

18. Wolfe F, Michaud K. Heart failure in rheumatoid arthritis: rates, predictors, and the effect of anti-tumor necrosis factor therapy. Am J Med 2004;116:305–11.

19. Nicola PJ, Maradit-Kremers H, Roger VL, et al. The risk of congestive heart failure in rheumatoid arthritis: a population-based study over 46 years. Arthritis Rheum 2005;52(2):412–20.

20. Myasoedova E, Crowson CS, Nicola PJ, et al. The influence of rheumatoid arthritis disease characteristics on heart failure. J Rheumatol 2011;38(8): 1601–6.

21. Mustonen J, Laakso M, Hirvonen T, et al. Abnormalities in left ventricular diastolic function in male patients with rheumatoid arthritis without clinically evident cardiovascular disease. Eur J Clin Invest 1993;23:246–53.

22. Crowson CS, Myasoedova E, Davis JM III, et al. Use of B-type natriuretic peptide as a screening tool for left ventricular diastolic dysfunction in rheumatoid

arthritis patients without clinical cardiovascular disease. Arthritis Care Res (Hoboken) 2011;63:729–34.

23. Corrao S, Sallì L, Arnone S, et al. Echo-Doppler left ventricular filling abnormalities in patients with rheumatoid arthritis without clinically evident cardiovascular disease. Eur J Clin Invest 1996;26(4):293–7.

24. Rudominer RL, Roman MJ, Devereux RB, et al. Independent association of rheumatoid arthritis with increased left ventricular mass but not with reduced ejection fraction. Arthritis Rheum 2009;60:22–9.

25. Yazici D, Tokay S, Aydin S, et al. Echocardiographic evaluation of cardiac diastolic function in patients with rheumatoid arthritis: 5 years of follow-up. Clin Rheumatol 2008;27:647–50.

26. Liang KP, Myasoedova E, Crowson CS, et al. Increased prevalence of diastolic dysfunction in rheumatoid arthritis. Ann Rheum Dis 2010;69(9):1665–70.

27. Gonzalez-Juanatey C, Testa A, Garcia-Castelo A, et al. Echocardiographic and Doppler findings in long-term treated rheumatoid arthritis patients without clinically evident cardiovascular disease. Semin Arthritis Rheum 2004;33(4): 231–8.

28. Aslam F, Bandeali S, Khan N, et al. Diastolic dysfunction in rheumatoid arthritis. A meta-analysis and systematic review. Arthritis Care Res 2013;65:534–43.

29. Correa de Sa DD, Hodge DO, Slusser JP, et al. Progression of preclinical diastolic dysfunction to the development of symptoms. Heart 2010;96:528–32.

30. Corrao S, Scaglione R, Calvo L, et al. A meta-analysis of the effect size of rheumatoid arthritis on left ventricular mass: comment on the article by Rudominer et al. Arthritis Rheum 2009;60(9):2851–2.

31. Giles JT, Malayeri AA, Fernandes V, et al. Left ventricular structure and function in patients with rheumatoid arthritis, as assessed by cardiac magnetic resonance imaging. Arthritis Rheum 2010;62(4):940–51.

32. Davis J, Knutson K, Strausbauch M, et al. Signature of aberrant immune responsiveness identifies myocardial dysfunction in rheumatoid arthritis. Arthritis Rheum 2011;63(6):1497–506.

33. Giles JT, Fert-Bober J, Park JK, et al. Myocardial citrullination in rheumatoid arthritis: a correlative histopathologic study. Arthritis Res Ther 2012;14(1):R39.

34. Costedoat-Chalumeau N, Hulot JS, Amoura Z, et al. Cardiomyopathy related to antimalarial therapy with illustrative case report. Cardiology 2007;107(2):73–80.

35. Nord JE, Shah PK, Rinaldi RZ, et al. Hydroxychloroquine cardiotoxicity in systemic lupus erythematosus: a report of 2 cases and review of the literature. Semin Arthritis Rheum 2004;33:336–51.

36. Cotroneo J, Sleik KM, Rene Rodriguez E, et al. Hydroxychloroquine-induced restrictive cardiomyopathy. Eur J Echocardiogr 2007;8:247–51.

37. Manohar VA, Moder KG, Edwards WD, et al. Restrictive cardiomyopathy secondary to hydroxychloroquine therapy. J Rheumatol 2009;36:440–1.

38. Muthukrishnan P, Roukoz H, Grafton G, et al. Hydroxychloroquine-induced cardiomyopathy: a case report. Circ Heart Fail 2011;4:e7–8.

39. Newton-Cheh C, Lin AE, Baggish AL, et al. Case records of the Massachusetts General Hospital. Case 11-2011. A 47-year-old man with systemic lupus erythematosus and heart failure. N Engl J Med 2011;364:1450–60.

40. Hartmann M, Meek IL, van Houwelingen GK, et al. Acute left ventricular failure in a patient with hydroxychloroquine-induced cardiomyopathy. Neth Heart J 2011; 19:482–5.

41. Azimian M, Gultekin SH, Hata JL, et al. Fatal antimalarial-induced cardiomyopathy: report of 2 cases. J Clin Rheumatol 2012;18(7):363–6.

42. Joyce E, Fabre A, Mahon N. Hydroxychloroquine cardiotoxicity presenting as a rapidly evolving biventricular cardiomyopathy. Eur Heart J Acute Cardiovasc Care 2013;2:77.

43. Sumpter MD, Tatro LS, Stoecker WV, et al. Evidence for risk of cardiomyopathy with hydroxychloroquine. Lupus 2012;21(14):1594–6.

44. Freihage JH, Patel NC, Jacobs WR, et al. Heart transplantation in a patient with chloroquine-induced cardiomyopathy. J Heart Lung Transplant 2004;23: 252–5.

45. Levine B, Kalman J, Mayer L, et al. Elevated circulating levels of tumor necrosis factor in severe chronic heart failure. N Engl J Med 1990;323:236–41.

46. Kadokami T, Frye C, Lemster B, et al. Anti-tumor necrosis factor-{alpha} antibody limits heart failure in a transgenic model. Circulation 2001;104:1094–7.

47. Li YY, Feng YQ, Kadokami T, et al. Myocardial extracellular matrix remodeling in transgenic mice overexpressing tumor necrosis factor alpha can be modulated by anti-tumor necrosis factor alpha therapy. Proc Natl Acad Sci U S A 2000;97: 12746–51.

48. Deswal A, Bozkurt B, Seta Y, et al. A phase I trial of tumor necrosis factor receptor (p75) fusion protein (TNFR: Fc) in patients with advanced heart failure. Circulation 1999;99:3224–6.

49. Mann DL, McMurray JJ, Packer M, et al. Targeted anticytokine therapy in patients with chronic heart failure: results of the Randomized Etanercept Worldwide Evaluation (RENEWAL). Circulation 2004;109:1594–602.

50. Chung ES, Packer M, Lo KH, et al, Anti-TNF therapy against congestive Heart Failure Investigators. Randomized, double-blind, placebo-controlled, pilot trial of infliximab, a chimeric monoclonal antibody to tumor necrosis factor-alpha, in patients with moderate-to-severe heart failure: results of the anti-TNF Therapy Against Congestive Heart Failure (ATTACH) trial. Circulation 2003;107(25): 3133–40.

51. Kwon HJ, Cote TR, Cuffe MS, et al. Case reports of heart failure after therapy with a tumor necrosis factor antagonist. Ann Intern Med 2003;138:807–11.

52. Jacobsson LT, Turesson C, Gülfe A, et al. Treatment with tumor necrosis factor blockers is associated with a lower incidence of first cardiovascular events in patients with rheumatoid arthritis. J Rheumatol 2005;32:1213–8.

53. Dixon WG, Watson KD, Lunt M, et al. Reduction in the incidence of myocardial infarction in patients with rheumatoid arthritis who respond to anti-tumor necrosis factor alpha therapy: results from the British Society for Rheumatology Biologics Register. Arthritis Rheum 2007;56:2905–12.

54. Carmona L, Descalzo MA, Perez-Pampin E, et al. All-cause and cause-specific mortality in rheumatoid arthritis are not greater than expected when treated with tumour necrosis factor antagonists. Ann Rheum Dis 2007;66:880–5.

55. Listing J, Strangfeld A, Kekow J, et al. Does tumor necrosis factor alpha inhibition promote or prevent heart failure in patients with rheumatoid arthritis? Arthritis Rheum 2008;58:667–77.

56. Cole J, Busti A, Kazi S. The incidence of new onset congestive heart failure and heart failure exacerbation in Veteran's Affairs patients receiving tumor necrosis factor α antagonists. Rheumatol Int 2007;27:369–73.

57. Barnabe C, Martin B, Ghali W. Systematic review and meta-analysis: anti-tumor necrosis factor α therapy and cardiovascular events in rheumatoid arthritis. Arthritis Care Res 2011;4:522–9.

58. Bely M, Apathy A. Amyloid A deposition in rheumatoid arthritis: a retrospective clinicopathologic study of 161 autopsy patients. Amyloid 2012;19(4):212–3.

59. Koivuniemi R, Paimela L, Suomalainen R, et al. Amyloidosis is frequently unde-tected in patients with rheumatoid. Amyloid 2008;15(4):262–8.
60. El Mansoury TM, Hazenberg BP, El Badawy SA, et al. Screening for amyloid in subcutaneous fat tissue of Egyptian patients with rheumatoid arthritis: clinical and laboratory characteristics. Ann Rheum Dis 2002;61:42–7.
61. Kuroda T, Tanabe N, Sakatsume M, et al. Comparison of gastroduodenal, renal and abdominal fat biopsies for diagnosing amyloidosis in rheumatoid arthritis. Clin Rheumatol 2002;21:123–8.
62. Kuroda T, Tanabe N, Kobayashi D, et al. Treatment with biologic agents im-proves the prognosis of patients with rheumatoid arthritis and amyloidosis. J Rheumatol 2012;39(7):1348–54.
63. Kuroda T, Wada Y, Kobayashi D, et al. Effective anti-TNF-alpha therapy can induce rapid resolution and sustained decrease of gastroduodenal mucosala-myloid deposits in reactive amyloidosis associated with rheumatoid arthritis. J Rheumatol 2009;36(11):2409–15.
64. Cruickshank B. Heart lesions in rheumatoid disease. J Pathol Bacteriol 1958;76: 223–40.
65. Lebowitz WB. The heart in rheumatoid arthritis: a clinical and pathological study of 62 cases. Ann Intern Med 1963;58:102–23.
66. van Albada-Kuipers GA, Bruijn JA, Westedt ML, et al. Coronary arteritis compli-cating rheumatoid arthritis. Ann Rheum Dis 1986;45(11):963–5.
67. Avina-Zubieta J, Thomas J, Sadatsafavi M, et al. Risk of incident cardiovascular events in patients with rheumatoid arthritis: a meta-analysis of observational studies. Ann Rheum Dis 2012;71:1524–9.
68. Douglas KM, Pace AV, Treharne GJ, et al. Excess recurrent cardiac events in rheumatoid arthritis patients with acute coronary syndrome. Ann Rheum Dis 2006;65(3):348–53.
69. Van Doornum S, Brand C, King B, et al. Increased case fatality rates following a first acute cardiovascular event in patients with rheumatoid arthritis. Arthritis Rheum 2006;54(7):2061–8.
70. Pasceri V, Yeh ET. A tale of two diseases: atherosclerosis and rheumatoid arthritis. Circulation 1999;100(21):2124–6.
71. Myasoedova E, Crowson CS, Kremers HM, et al. Total cholesterol and LDL levels decrease before rheumatoid arthritis. Ann Rheum Dis 2010;69:1310–4.
72. Myasoedova E, Crowson C, Kremers H, et al. Lipid paradox in rheumatoid arthritis: the impact of serum lipid measures and systemic inflammation on the risk of cardiovascular disease. Ann Rheum Dis 2011;70(3):482–7.
73. Hahn BH, Grossman J, Ansell BJ, et al. Altered lipoprotein metabolism in chronic inflammatory states: proinflammatory high-density lipoprotein and accelerated atherosclerosis in systemic lupus erythematosus and rheumatoid arthritis. Arthritis Res Ther 2008;10(4):213.
74. Charles-Schoeman C, Watanabe J, Lee YY, et al. Abnormal function of high den-sity lipoprotein is associated with poor disease control and an altered protein cargo in rheumatoid arthritis. Arthritis Rheum 2009;60(10):2870–9.
75. Wada Y, Kuroda T, Murasawa A, et al. Autoantibodies against oxidized low-density lipoprotein (LDL) and carotid atherosclerosis in patients with rheumatoid arthritis. Clin Exp Rheumatol 2005;23:482–6.
76. Hurt-Camejo E, Paredes S, Masana L, et al. Elevated levels of small, low-density lipoprotein with high affinity for arterial matrix components in patients with rheu-matoid arthritis: possible contribution of phospholipase A2 to this atherogenic profile. Arthritis Rheum 2001;44:2761–7.

77. Dursunoğlu D, Evrengül H, Polat B, et al. Lp(a) lipoprotein and lipids in patients with rheumatoid arthritis: serum levels and relationship to inflammation. Rheumatol Int 2005;25(4):241–5.

78. Park YB, Choi HK, Kim MY, et al. Effects of antirheumatic therapy on serum lipid levels in patients with rheumatoid arthritis: a prospective study. Am J Med 2002; 113:188–93.

79. Boers M, Nurmohamed MT, Doelman CJ, et al. Influence of glucocorticoids and disease activity on total and high density lipoprotein cholesterol in patients with rheumatoid arthritis. Ann Rheum Dis 2003;62:842–5.

80. Morris S, Wasko M, Antohe J, et al. Hydroxychloroquine use associated with improvement in lipid profiles in rheumatoid arthritis patients. Arthritis Care Res 2011;63(4):530–4.

81. van Sijl AM, Peters MJ, Knol DL, et al. The effect of TNF-α blocking therapy on lipid levels in rheumatoid arthritis: a meta-analysis. Semin Arthritis Rheum 2011; 41(3):393–400.

82. Jones G, Sebba A, Gu J, et al. Comparison of tocilizumab monotherapy versus methotrexate monotherapy in patients with moderate to severe rheumatoid arthritis: the AMBITION study. Ann Rheum Dis 2010;69:88–96.

83. Maini RN, Taylor PC, Szechinski J, et al. Double-blind randomized controlled clinical trial of the interleukin-6 receptor antagonist, tocilizumab, in European patients with rheumatoid arthritis who had an incomplete response to methotrexate. Arthritis Rheum 2006;54:2817–9.

84. Schiff MH, Kremer JM, Jahreis A, et al. Integrated safety in tocilizumab clinical trials. Arthritis Res Ther 2011;13(5):R141.

85. Weinblatt ME, Kremer J, Cush J, et al. Tocilizumab as monotherapy or in combination with nonbiologic disease-modifying antirheumatic drugs: twenty-four-week results of an open-label, clinical practice study. Arthritis Care Res 2013; 65(3):362–71.

86. Genovese MC, Sebba A, Rubbert-Roth A, et al. Long-term safety of tocilizumab in rheumatoid arthritis clinical trials. Presented at ACR [abstract 2217]. Chicago, 2011.

87. Fleischmann R, Kremer J, Cush J, et al. Placebo-controlled trial of tofacitinib monotherapy in rheumatoid arthritis. N Engl J Med 2012;367:495–507.

88. van Vollenhoven RF, Fleischmann R, Cohen S, et al. Tofacitinib or adalimumab versus placebo in rheumatoid arthritis. N Engl J Med 2012;367:508–19.

89. Burmester GR, Blanco R, Charles-Schoeman C, et al. Tofacitinib (CP-690,550) in combination with methotrexate in patients with active rheumatoid arthritis with an inadequate response to tumour necrosis factor inhibitors: a randomised phase 3 trial. Lancet 2013;381(9865):451–60.

90. McCarey DW, McInnes IB, Madhok R, et al. Trial of Atorvastatin in Rheumatoid Arthritis (TARA): double-blind, randomized placebo-controlled trial. Lancet 2004;363:2015–21.

91. Sheng X, Murphy MJ, Macdonald TM, et al. Effectiveness of statins on total cholesterol and cardiovascular disease and all-cause mortality in osteoarthritis and rheumatoid arthritis. J Rheumatol 2012;39:32–40.

92. Cojocaru L, Rusali AC, Suţa C, et al. The role of simvastatin in the therapeutic approach of rheumatoid arthritis. Autoimmune Dis 2013;2013:326258.

93. Van Doornum S, McColl G, Wicks IP. Atorvastatin reduces arterial stiffness in patients with rheumatoid arthritis. Ann Rheum Dis 2004;63(12):1571–5.

94. Hermann F, Forster A, Chenevard R, et al. Simvastatin improves endothelial function in patients with rheumatoid arthritis. J Am Coll Cardiol 2005;45(3):461–4.

95. Maki-Petaja KM, Booth AD, Hall FC, et al. Ezetimibe and simvastatin reduce inflammation, disease activity, and aortic stiffness and improve endothelial function in rheumatoid arthritis. J Am Coll Cardiol 2007;50(9):852–8.
96. De Vera MA, Choi H, Abrahamowicz M, et al. Statin discontinuation and risk of acute myocardial infarction in patients with rheumatoid arthritis: a population-based cohort study. Ann Rheum Dis 2011;70:1020–4.
97. Panoulas V, Douglas K, Milionis H, et al. Prevalence and associations of hypertension and its control in patients with rheumatoid arthritis. Rheumatology (Oxford) 2007;46:1477–82.
98. Boyer JF, Gourraud PA, Cantagrel A, et al. Traditional cardiovascular risk factors in rheumatoid arthritis: a meta-analysis. Joint Bone Spine 2012;78:179–83.
99. Chung C, Giles J, Petri M, et al. Prevalence of traditional modifiable cardiovascular risk factors in patients with rheumatoid arthritis: comparison with control subjects from the multi-ethnic study of atherosclerosis. Semin Arthritis Rheum 2012;41:535–44.
100. Han C, Robinson D, Hackett M, et al. Cardiovascular disease and risk factors in patients with rheumatoid arthritis, psoriatic arthritis, and ankylosing spondylitis. J Rheumatol 2006;33:2167–72.
101. Simard J, Mittleman M. Prevalent rheumatoid arthritis and diabetes among NHANES III participants aged 60 and older. J Rheumatol 2007;34:469–73.
102. Solomon D, Curhan G, Rimm E, et al. Cardiovascular risk factors in women with and without rheumatoid arthritis. Arthritis Rheum 2004;50:3444–9.
103. La Montagna G, Cacciapuoti F, Buono R, et al. Insulin resistance is an independent risk factor for atherosclerosis in rheumatoid arthritis. Diab Vasc Dis Res 2007;4(2):130–5.
104. Chung CP, Oeser A, Solus JF, et al. Prevalence of the metabolic syndrome is increased in rheumatoid arthritis and is associated with coronary atherosclerosis. Atherosclerosis 2008;196(2):756–63.
105. Dessein P, Joffe B, Stanwix A. Inflammation, insulin resistance, and aberrant lipid metabolism as cardiovascular risk factors in rheumatoid arthritis. J Rheumatol 2003;30(7):1403–5.
106. Hotamisligil GS, Arner P, Caro JF, et al. Increased adipose tissue expression of tumor necrosis factor-alpha in human obesity and insulin resistance. J Clin Invest 1995;95(5):2409–15.
107. Kern PA, Saghizadeh M, Ong JM, et al. The expression of tumor necrosis factor in human adipose tissue. Regulation by obesity, weight loss, and relationship to lipoprotein lipase. J Clin Invest 1995;95(5):2111–9.
108. Saghizadeh M, Ong JM, Garvey WT, et al. The expression of TNF alpha by human muscle. Relationship to insulin resistance. J Clin Invest 1996;97(4):1111–6.
109. Hotamisligil GS, Murray DL, Choy LN, et al. Tumor necrosis factor alpha inhibits signaling from the insulin receptor. Proc Natl Acad Sci USA 1994;91:4854–8.
110. Nilsson J, Jovinge S, Niemann A, et al. Relation between plasma tumor necrosis factor-alpha and insulin sensitivity in elderly men with non-insulin-dependent diabetes mellitus. Arterioscler Thromb Vasc Biol 1998;18(8):1199–202.
111. Peters MJ, van Halm VP, Voskuyl AE, et al. Does rheumatoid arthritis equal diabetes mellitus as an independent risk factor for cardiovascular disease? A prospective study. Arthritis Rheum 2009;61:1571–9.
112. Crowson CS, Therneau TM, Davis JM 3rd, et al. Brief report: accelerated aging influences cardiovascular disease risk in rheumatoid arthritis. Arthritis Rheum 2013;65(10):2562–6.

113. Maradit-Kremers HM, Nicola PJ, Crowson CS, et al. Prognostic importance of low body mass index in relation to cardiovascular mortality in rheumatoid arthritis. Arthritis Rheum 2004;50(11):3450–7.
114. George J, Levy Y, Shoenfeld Y. Smoking and immunity: an additional player in the mosaic of autoimmunity. Scand J Immunol 1997;45:1–6.
115. Costenbader K, Feskanich D, Mandl L, et al. Smoking intensity, duration, and cessation, and the risk of rheumatoid arthritis in women. Am J Med 2006;119:503–9.
116. Saag K, Cerhan J, Kolluri S, et al. Cigarette smoking and rheumatoid arthritis severity. Ann Rheum Dis 1997;56:463–9.
117. Helmersson J, Larsson A, Vessby B, et al. Active smoking and a history of smoking are associated with enhanced prostaglandin F(2alpha), interleukin-6 and F2-isoprostane formation in elderly men. Atherosclerosis 2005;181:201–7.
118. Gerli R, Sherer Y, Vaudo G, et al. Early atherosclerosis in rheumatoid arthritis: effect of smoking on thickness of the carotid artery intima media. Ann N Y Acad Sci 2005;1051:281–90.
119. Maradit-Kremers H, Crowson CS, Therneau TM, et al. High ten year risk of cardiovascular disease in newly diagnosed rheumatoid arthritis patients. Arthritis Rheum 2008;58:2268–74.
120. Young A, Koduri G, Batley M, et al. Mortality in rheumatoid arthritis. Increased in the early course of disease, in ischaemic heart disease and in pulmonary fibrosis. Rheumatology 2007;46:350–7.
121. Goodson NJ, Wiles NJ, Lunt M, et al. Mortality in early inflammatory polyarthritis: cardiovascular mortality is increased in seropositive patients. Arthritis Rheum 2002;46:2010–9.
122. Georgiadis AN, Voulgari PV, Argyropoulou MI, et al. Early treatment reduces the cardiovascular risk factors in newly diagnosed rheumatoid arthritis patients. Semin Arthritis Rheum 2008;38:13–9.
123. Hannawi S, Haluska B, Marwick T, et al. Atherosclerotic disease is increased in recent-onset rheumatoid arthritis: a critical role for inflammation. Arthritis Res Ther 2007;9:R116.
124. Kao AH, Krishnaswami S, Cunningham A, et al. Subclinical coronary artery calcification and relationship to disease duration in women with rheumatoid arthritis. J Rheumatol 2008;35(1):61–9.
125. Chung CP, Oeser A, Raggi P, et al. Increased coronary-artery atherosclerosis in rheumatoid arthritis: relationship to disease duration and cardiovascular risk factors. Arthritis Rheum 2005;52(10):3045–53.
126. Turesson C, Jacobsson LT, Sturfelt G, et al. Rheumatoid factor and antibodies to cyclic citrullinated peptides are associated with severe extra-articular manifestations in rheumatoid arthritis. Ann Rheum Dis 2007;66:59–64.
127. Sihvonen S, Korpela M, Mustila A, et al. The predictive value of rheumatoid factor isotypes, anti-cyclic citrullinated peptide antibodies and antineutrophil cytoplasmic antibodies for mortality in patients with rheumatoid arthritis. J Rheumatol 2005;32(11):2089–94.
128. Gerli R, Bartolini Bocci E, Sherer Y, et al. Association of anti-cyclic citrullinated peptide antibodies with subclinical atherosclerosis in patients with rheumatoid arthritis. Ann Rheum Dis 2008;67:724–5.
129. Farragher TM, Goodson NJ, Naseem H, et al. Association of the HLA-DRB1 gene with premature death, particularly from cardiovascular disease, in patients with rheumatoid arthritis and inflammatory polyarthritis. Arthritis Rheum 2008;58:359–69.

130. Mattey DL, Thomson W, Ollier W, et al. Association of DRB1 shared epitope geno-types with early mortality in rheumatoid arthritis: results of eighteen years of fol-lowup from the early rheumatoid arthritis study. Arthritis Rheum 2007;56:1408–16.
131. Gonzalez-Gay MA, Gonzalez-Juanatey C, Lopez-Diaz MJ, et al. HLA-DRB1 and persistent chronic inflammation contribute to cardiovascular events and cardio-vascular mortality in patients with rheumatoid arthritis. Arthritis Rheum 2007;57: 125–32.
132. Goodson NJ, Symmons DP, Scott DG, et al. Baseline levels of C-reactive protein and prediction of death from cardiovascular disease in patients with inflamma-tory polyarthritis: a ten-year followup study of a primary care-based inception cohort. Arthritis Rheum 2005;52:2293–9.
133. Graf J, Scherzer R, Grunfeld C, et al. Levels of C-reactive protein associated with high and very high cardiovascular risk are prevalent in patients with rheu-matoid arthritis. PLoS One 2009;4:e6242.
134. Gonzalez-Gay MA, Gonzalez-Juanatey C, Pineiro A, et al. High-grade C-reac-tive protein elevation correlates with accelerated atherogenesis in patients with rheumatoid arthritis. J Rheumatol 2005;32(7):1219–23.
135. Libby P. Inflammation and cardiovascular disease mechanisms. Am J Clin Nutr 2006;83:456S–60S.
136. Fonseca JE, Santos MJ, Canhão H, et al. Interleukin-6 as a key player in sys-temic inflammation and joint destruction. Autoimmun Rev 2009;8:538–42.
137. Schieffer B, Schieffer E, Hilfiker-Kleiner D, et al. Expression of angiotensin II and interleukin 6 in human coronary atherosclerotic plaques: potential implications for inflammation and plaque instability. Circulation 2000;101:1372–8.
138. Olopien B, Hyper M, Kowalski J, et al. A new immunological marker of athero-sclerotic injury of arterial wall. Res Commun Mol Pathol Pharmacol 2001;109: 241–8.
139. Cesari M, Penninx BW, Newman AB, et al. Inflammatory markers and onset of cardiovascular events: results from the health ABC study. Circulation 2003; 108:2317–22.
140. Barath P, Fishbein MC, Cao J, et al. Detection and localization of tumor necrosis factor in human atheroma. Am J Cardiol 1990;65:297–302.
141. Schjerning Olsen AM, Fosbøl EL, Lindhardsen J, et al. Duration of treatment with nonsteroidal anti-inflammatory drugs and impact on risk of death and recurrent myocardial infarction in patients with prior myocardial infarction: a nationwide cohort study. Circulation 2011;123(20):2226–35.
142. Trelle S, Reichenbach S, Wandel S, et al. Cardiovascular safety of non-steroidal anti-inflammatory drugs: network meta-analysis. BMJ 2011;342:c7086.
143. Hudson M, Baron M, Rahme E, et al. Ibuprofen may abrogate the benefits of aspirin when used for secondary prevention of myocardial infarction. J Rheumatol 2005;32(8):1589–93.
144. Goodson NJ, Brookhart AM, Symmons DP, et al. Nonsteroidal anti-inflammatory drug use does not appear to be associated with increased cardiovascular mor-tality in patients with inflammatory polyarthritis: results from a primary care based inception cohort of patients. Ann Rheum Dis 2009;68:367–72.
145. Lindhardsen J, Gislason GH, Jacobsen S, et al. Non-steroidal anti-inflammatory drugs and risk of cardiovascular disease in patients with rheumatoid arthritis: a nationwide cohort study. Ann Rheum Dis 2013. [Epub ahead of print].
146. Wei L, MacDonald TM, Walker BR. Taking glucocorticoids by prescription is associated with subsequent cardiovascular disease. Ann Intern Med 2004; 141:764–70.

147. Greenberg J, Kremer J, Curtis J, et al. Tumor necrosis factor antagonist use and associated risk reduction of cardiovascular events among patients with rheumatoid arthritis. Ann Rheum Dis 2011;70:576–82.

148. Davis JM III, Maradit Kremers H, Crowson CS, et al. Glucocorticoids and cardiovascular events in rheumatoid arthritis: a population-based cohort study. Arthritis Rheum 2007;56:820–30.

149. Aviña-Zubieta JA, Abrahamowicz M, De Vera MA, et al. Immediate and past cumulative effects of oral glucocorticoids on the risk of acute myocardial infarction in rheumatoid arthritis: a population-based study. Rheumatology (Oxford) 2013;52(1):68–75.

150. Aviña-Zubieta JA, Abrahamowicz M, Choi HK, et al. Risk of cerebrovascular disease associated with the use of glucocorticoids in patients with incident rheumatoid arthritis: a population-based study. Ann Rheum Dis 2011;70(6):990–5.

151. Crowson CS, Matteson EL, Roger VL, et al. Usefulness of risk scores to estimate the risk of cardiovascular disease in patients with rheumatoid arthritis. Am J Cardiol 2012;110(3):420–4.

152. Peters MJ, Symmons DP, McCarey D, et al. EULAR evidence-based recommendations for cardiovascular risk management in patients with rheumatoid arthritis and other forms of inflammatory arthritis. Ann Rheum Dis 2010;69:325–31.

153. Crowson C, Gabriel S. Towards improving cardiovascular risk management in patients with RA: need for a accurate risk assessment. Ann Rheum Dis 2011; 70:719–21.

154. Toms TE, Panoulas VF, Douglas KM, et al. Statin use in rheumatoid arthritis in relation to actual cardiovascular risk: evidence for substantial under treatment of lipid associated cardiovascular risk? Ann Rheum Dis 2010;69:683–8.

155. Tikiz C, Utuk O, Pirildar T, et al. Effects of angiotensin-converting enzyme inhibition and statin treatment on inflammatory markers and endothelial functions in patients with longterm rheumatoid arthritis. J Rheumatol 2005;32: 2095–101.

156. Flammer AJ, Sudano I, Hermann F, et al. Angiotensin-converting enzyme inhibition improves vascular function in rheumatoid arthritis. Circulation 2008;117: 2262–9.

157. Martin MF, Surrall KE, McKenna F, et al. Captopril: a new treatment for rheumatoid arthritis? Lancet 1984;1:1325–8.

158. Choi HK, Hernan MA, Seeger JD, et al. Methotrexate and mortality in patients with rheumatoid arthritis: a prospective study. Lancet 2002;359:1173–7.

159. Westlake SL, Colebatch AN, Baird J, et al. The effect of methotrexate on cardiovascular disease in patients with rheumatoid arthritis: a systematic literature review. Rheumatology (Oxford) 2010;49:295–307.

160. Micha R, Imamura F, Wyler von Ballmoos M, et al. Systematic review and meta-analysis of methotrexate use and risk of cardiovascular disease. Am J Cardiol 2011;108:1362–70.

161. El-Barbary A, Kassem E, El-Sergany MA, et al. Association of anti-modified citrullinated vimentin with subclinical atherosclerosis in early rheumatoid arthritis compared with anti-cyclic citrullinated peptide. J Rheumatol 2011;38(5):828–34.

162. Solomon DH, Curtis JR, Saag KG, et al. Cardiovascular risk in rheumatoid arthritis: comparing TNF-α blockade with nonbiologic DMARDs. Am J Med 2013;126(8):730.e9–17.

163. Al-Aly Z, Pan H, Zeringue A, et al. Tumor necrosis factor-alpha blockade, cardiovascular outcomes, and survival in rheumatoid arthritis. Transl Res 2011;157: 10–8.

164. Provan SA, Semb AG, Hisdal J, et al. Remission is the goal for cardiovascular risk management in patients with rheumatoid arthritis: a cross-sectional comparative study. Ann Rheum Dis 2011;70:812–7.
165. Maki-Petaja KM, Hall FC, Booth AD, et al. Rheumatoid arthritis is associated with increased aortic pulse-wave velocity, which is reduced by anti-tumor necrosis factor-alpha therapy. Circulation 2006;114:1185–92.
166. Galarraga B, Khan F, Kumar P, et al. Etanercept improves inflammation-associated arterial stiffness in rheumatoid arthritis. Rheumatology (Oxford) 2009;48:1418–23.
167. Wong M, Oakley SP, Young L, et al. Infliximab improves vascular stiffness in patients with rheumatoid arthritis. Ann Rheum Dis 2009;68:1277–84.
168. Barnabe C, Martin BJ, Ghali WA. Systematic review and meta-analysis: anti-tumor necrosis factor alpha therapy and cardiovascular events in rheumatoid arthritis. Arthritis Care Res (Hoboken) 2011;63:522–9.

Cardiac Manifestations of Systemic Lupus Erythematosus

Jonathan J. Miner, MD, PhD, Alfred H.J. Kim, MD, PhD*

KEYWORDS

- Systemic lupus erythematosus • Neonatal lupus • Congenital heart block
- Myocarditis • Pericarditis • Coronary artery disease • Libman-Sacks

KEY POINTS

- Systemic lupus erythematosus can affect any part of the heart.
- Cardiac manifestations of lupus include myocarditis, pericarditis, valvular disease, thrombosis, and cardiac conduction defects.
- Coronary artery disease is more common in patients with lupus.
- Congenital heart block occurs frequently as a result of maternal anti-Ro/SS-A antibodies.

NEONATAL LUPUS AND CONGENITAL HEART BLOCK

Autoantibodies serve as a diagnostic tool for systemic lupus erythematosus (SLE) and other autoimmune diseases, but certain autoantibodies are thought to be directly pathogenic in some circumstances. For example, the presence of anti-Ro/SS-A autoantibodies is strongly associated with the risk of developing neonatal lupus erythematosus as a form of passively transferred autoimmunity from mother to child.[1,2] Neonatal lupus is a congenital disorder in which the cardiac conduction system is often damaged by maternal anti-Ro/SS-A autoantibodies that cross the placenta.[1,2] Infants with neonatal lupus sometimes develop complete heart block, which requires pacing for survival. Complete heart block in the fetus is associated with fetal myocarditis.[3] Neonatal lupus can develop whenever a pregnant woman has circulating anti-Ro/SS-A antibodies, even if she does not have SLE. This possibility includes patients with Sjögren syndrome and even asymptomatic patients with anti-Ro/SS-A.[4] Studies have estimated that between 60% and 90% of all cases of congenital heart block are secondary to maternal autoantibodies that are transferred to the fetus across the placenta.[5,6]

Although anti-Ro/SS-A antibodies might be directly pathogenic to the fetus, adults with anti-Ro/SS-A are not prone to developing heart block. However, several recent studies have found evidence that the QTc interval is prolonged in adults with

Division of Rheumatology, Department of Medicine, Washington University School of Medicine, 660 South Euclid Avenue, Campus Box 8045, St Louis, MO 63110, USA
* Corresponding author.
E-mail address: akim@dom.wustl.edu

Rheum Dis Clin N Am 40 (2014) 51–60
http://dx.doi.org/10.1016/j.rdc.2013.10.003
0889-857X/14/$ – see front matter © 2014 Elsevier Inc. All rights reserved.

anti-Ro/SS-A and that certain ventricular arrhythmias may be more common in adults with these autoantibodies.[7–9] One study found a statistically significant difference in QTc interval, with anti-Ro/SS-A being associated with a mean QTc of 445 milliseconds compared with 419 milliseconds in patients lacking the autoantibody.[7] This finding suggests that anti-Ro/SS-A autoantibodies may contribute to a mild form of conduction disease in adults.

It is difficult to explain the discrepancy between neonatal and adult conduction disease. One hypothesis involves a contribution from an unknown fetal factor that enhances the effect of anti-Ro/SSA autoantibodies.[10] In support of this, immune complexes directed against the fetal conduction system have been observed.[11] However, only about 2% of fetuses develop congenital heart block in the presence of anti-Ro/SS-A antibodies.[12] Furthermore, epidemiologic studies do not directly support the presence of a pathogenic fetal factor. If a mother with anti-Ro/SS-A autoantibodies has had prior offspring with complete heart block, the probability of future offspring developing complete heart block increases from 2% to 18%.[13] However, monozygotic twins of mothers with circulating anti-Ro/SS-A antibodies discordantly develop congenital heart block,[14] which implies that the pathogenesis of neonatal complete heart block is complex and that it does not simply depend on the presence of anti-Ro/SS-A and an unknown fetal factor. An alternative hypothesis is that certain autoantibodies are destructive only to the developing cardiac conduction system, possibly because of exposure of unique antigens in the fetus, but monozygotic twin discordance makes this possibility less likely. In addition, small differences within the uterine environment or in the developing immune system might contribute to discordant phenotypes in genetically identical neonates,[15] but this has yet to be demonstrated.

Progression of incomplete heart block to irreversible complete heart block can sometimes be prevented by treatment with corticosteroids.[16] Some case reports describe postnatal progression of heart block despite depletion of circulating autoantibodies.[17] Given the severe, potentially life-threatening, complications of neonatal lupus, it is important to explain this risk to women of child-bearing age who are known to have anti-Ro/SSA antibodies. Maternal use of hydroxychloroquine may reduce the risk of recurrent neonatal lupus in subsequent pregnancies.[18]

PERICARDITIS

Pericarditis is the most common cardiac manifestation of SLE. Approximately 25% of all patients with SLE develop symptomatic pericarditis at some point during the course of the disease, most often along with associated pleuritis.[19,20] However, autopsy studies reveal a higher rate of subclinical pericarditis.[20] It is rare for pericarditis to be the only symptom at presentation.

Patients with lupus pericarditis typically present with tachycardia, substernal or precordial chest discomfort, dyspnea, and positional pain. Some patients may have a friction rub on examination. All of these signs and symptoms are typical of pericarditis in general. Echocardiographic findings (pericardial effusion and thickened pericardium) and electrocardiogram changes (PR depression and diffuse ST segment elevation) are also similar to other forms of pericarditis.

The conventional wisdom is that tamponade and constrictive pericarditis are rare in SLE. Constrictive pericarditis has only been reported in SLE in a few patients.[21,22] Tamponade is uncommon compared with the overall frequency of pericarditis in patients with lupus. For example, one large study of 1300 patients found tamponade in less than 1% of patients.[23] However, other retrospective studies have found between that 13% and 22% of patients with symptomatic pericarditis had evidence of tamponade, suggesting that it might be more common than previously appreciated.[24,25] Tamponade has also been reported as the initial, presenting manifestation of SLE.[26,27] Severe pericarditis and tamponade might be more likely to occur in patients when the diagnosis or treatment are delayed,[27] which could explain the differences in the prevalence of tamponade in various patient populations.

Pericardial fluid from patients with lupus pericarditis typically reveals inflammatory exudate with neutrophil predominance. Pericardial biopsy is not required to establish a diagnosis, but histopathology often reveals mononuclear cells, fibrinous material, and immune complex deposition.[28,29] Autoantibodies can sometimes be detected in the pericardial fluid,[29] although this is not diagnostically useful.

Whether to check antinuclear antibody (ANA) in patients with a first episode of pericarditis depends on the clinical situation. A positive ANA test is nonspecific and occurs frequently in patients who do not have SLE. Positive results are often confusing for patients and have poor predictive value when ordered inappropriately.[30] As a general rule, it is reasonable to check ANA in patients who have additional signs or symptoms of lupus or in those who have had recurrent, unexplained bouts of idiopathic pericarditis. The clinical context is important to consider. For example, patients with idiopathic pericarditis are more likely to have had a recent viral infection, whereas the presence of leukopenia and/or lymphopenia, Raynaud, or a malar rash suggests the possibility of SLE.

Mild pericarditis can be treated with nonsteroidal antiinflammatory drugs, but most patients with lupus pericarditis require corticosteroids in addition to optimization of disease-modifying antirheumatic drug (DMARD) therapy.[31] Selection of an appropriate DMARD depends on the severity of disease and whether the patient has additional organ-threatening disease. For example, a patient with tamponade and/or class IV nephritis requires high-dose corticosteroids in addition to cyclophosphamide or mycophenolate mofetil, whereas patients with mild- to-moderate disease may respond to a slow steroid taper combined with hydroxychloroquine, methotrexate, or azathioprine. Biologic DMARD therapies such as rituximab or belimumab have not been definitively shown to treat lupus pericarditis, although there is likely to be a role for these therapies in some patients.

MYOCARDITIS AND CARDIOMYOPATHY

Clinically apparent lupus myocarditis is rare.[32] As with pericarditis, autopsy studies have revealed subclinical myocarditis in a higher percentage of patients.[33] Autoimmune myocarditis with deposition of immune complexes has been shown at autopsy and by endomyocardial biopsy. Pathology typically reveals mononuclear cell infiltrates, perivascular inflammation or arteriopathy, and necrosis of the cardiomyocytes. The primary lesion is thought to be perivascular inflammation.[34] Patients with lupus myocarditis can present with symptoms of heart failure including resting tachycardia and dyspnea, but they also sometimes present with chest discomfort, fever, and/or myopericarditis. Global hypokinesis on echocardiogram in patients without evidence of coronary artery disease (CAD) supports the diagnosis. Cardiac magnetic resonance imaging (MRI) shows delayed gadolinium enhancement in lupus myocarditis, although it cannot always distinguish among the various forms of myocarditis.[35,36] Biopsy is typically low yield and not required for the diagnosis, although it can be helpful in some patients.[37] Treatment with high-dose methylprednisolone is typically required, as is optimization of DMARD therapy.

Advances in human genetics research have led to the identification of specific genes and mutations that appear to contribute to pathogenesis of SLE. For example, mutations in the DNA exonuclease Trex1 have been associated with SLE in approximately 2% to 3% of patients.[38,39] Mice lacking Trex1 develop a lupus-like disease with severe, fatal myocarditis.[40] This mouse model may continue to yield important insights into the pathogenesis of myocarditis in patients with SLE. In addition to myocarditis, some patients with SLE develop cardiomyopathy, which can be directly caused by the SLE. However, cardiomyopathy in SLE can also be secondary to CAD, which is common in patients with SLE.[41] Cardiomyopathy secondary to hydroxychloroquine has also been reported, although this is rare at doses typically prescribed for SLE.[42] The most common cause for cardiomyopathy in patients with SLE is likely coexisting hypertension and/or CAD. Cardiomyopathy secondary to small vessel disease and thrombosis of the microcirculation have also been described.[43]

Sometimes it is difficult to determine whether cardiomyopathy is secondary to lupus myocarditis or another underlying process. In addition to cardiac MRI, another useful diagnostic approach is to perform an echocardiographic or nuclear medicine evaluation for reversibility after a period of treatment with high-dose corticosteroids. However, patients with lupus with cardiomyopathy almost always require additional cardiac work-up to exclude other underlying causes, including an evaluation for underlying CAD.

CAD

During the second half of the twentieth century, CAD became an increasingly appreciated manifestation of SLE.[41,44,45] CAD is the most common cause of death in patients with late-onset or long-standing SLE.[41] In addition to CAD, there are also reports of other forms of coronary inflammation and thrombosis in patients with SLE.[46,47] These reports include examples of vasospasm, coronary arteritis, and embolization into coronary arteries. However, these phenomena are less common. Atherosclerosis remains the most prevalent and significant mortality risk in older adult patients with SLE.

Thrombosis and inflammation were once thought to be distinct, but over the last few decades it has become increasingly clear that these processes are linked. Several studies have described an association between antiphospholipid antibodies and development of CAD,[48] whereas others have failed to show an association. One group found that anticardiolipin antibody levels predicted atherosclerosis independently of other risk factors.[49]

The risk of fatal myocardial infarction increases with time from diagnosis with SLE,[44] but one of the most striking features of CAD in patients with lupus is the development of premature CAD. Even children with SLE have been noted to develop premature atherosclerosis, including 1 case of myocardial infarction in a 5-year-old patient.[50] Young women with SLE are at greater risk of developing myocardial infarction at an early age, even when controlling for other risk factors.[51] However, not all patients with lupus seem to have similar susceptibility to developing premature atherosclerosis. There is no reliable method for predicting the patients who are at the greatest risk, but it is reasonable to assume that patients with traditional risk factors like hypertension, a history of smoking, a family history of CAD, and hyperlipidemia have higher risk. Markers of inflammation predict cardiovascular risk,[52] and therefore systemic inflammation is likely to be driving premature atherosclerosis. It is not known whether improved control of systemic inflammation could have an impact on the frequency of cardiovascular events in patients with SLE.

Treatment with corticosteroids increases the risk of developing CAD by contributing to hyperlipidemia, hypertension, weight gain, and the development of steroid-induced diabetes mellitus. However, high-density lipoprotein levels are lower in patients with lupus even in the absence of corticosteroid therapy.[53] Petri and colleagues[54] found that an increase in prednisone of 10 mg per day results in an average increase of 2.5 kg in weight, a 1.1 mm Hg increase in blood pressure, and a 7.5 mg/dL increase in total cholesterol. Longer duration of corticosteroid therapy increases the risk of developing subclinical cardiovascular disease and independently predicts risk of cardiovascular events. Another study found that patients on 30 mg of prednisone daily have a 60% greater 2-year risk of cardiovascular events compared with patients with lupus with the same risk factors and disease activity but not taking corticosteroids.[55] This finding further underscores the importance of minimizing corticosteroid dose whenever possible.

Patients with SLE are more likely to have subclinical CAD.[56] When young patients with lupus complain of chest pain, myocardial infarction ought to remain in the differential diagnosis even when it would be easily dismissed in patients lacking more traditional risk factors. Because of the increased risk of atherosclerosis in patients with lupus, a reasonable preventative approach is to have a lower threshold for initiation of statin therapy, a lower target low-density lipoprotein, and lower blood pressure goal (130/80 mm Hg). Patients with chronic, systemic inflammation are increasingly being classified as having a CAD risk equivalent,[57] much like patients with diabetes mellitus. Hydroxychloroquine is associated with favorable effects on lipids and blood glucose,[58] and so it might reduce the risk of cardiovascular events. The reduction in cardiovascular disease activity by lipid-lowering therapy seen in patients who do not have SLE (including those with rheumatoid arthritis or multiple sclerosis) has not been realized in patients with SLE. In a placebo-controlled study where 200 adults with SLE were randomized to receive atorvastatin or placebo, no differences were observed in coronary artery calcium, carotid intima media thickness, carotid plaque, SLE disease activity, or endothelial cell activation.[59]

As with SLE, rheumatoid arthritis (RA) causes premature atherosclerosis, leading to increased mortality caused by myocardial infarction. Autopsies of patients with RA revealed that their atherosclerotic plaques were more likely to contain a thin, inflamed fibrous cap that is especially prone to rupture and myocardial infarction.[60] Although this issue still needs additional investigation, a recent study suggested that carotid atherosclerotic plaques in patients with lupus seem to be more vulnerable based on echolucency.[61] Because inflammation promotes plaque rupture,[62] it puts these patients at greater risk.

VALVULAR DISEASE

In 1924, Libman and Sacks[63] reported "atypical verrucous endocarditis" in four patients. This observation is generally regarded as the first description of lupus-associated sterile endocarditis, also known as Libman-Sacks endocarditis. Two of the four reported patients had a malar rash, and all four had other features suggesting systemic lupus, including evidence of pericarditis.[63] Estimates of the prevalence of Libman-Sacks endocarditis in SLE patients range from 11% to 74%.[64] Libman-Sacks most commonly affects the mitral valve, although any valve can be involved. Transesophageal echocardiogram is the most useful method for detecting valvular disease.[65] The fibrinous lesions contain inflammatory cells and have only rarely been reported to embolize. Clinically significant valvular dysfunction secondary to Libman-Sacks endocarditis is not common, occurring in just 1% to 2% of patients according to one study.[66] However, another prospective study suggested a higher incidence of clinically significant valvular disease in up to 18% of patients.[20] Only patients with especially large valvular lesions might require anticoagulation. High-dose cortico-steroids have also been used to treat large lesions once infection has been excluded, but the evidence for this treatment is still inconclusive. Valvular disease severe enough to require valve replacement is less common.[67]

Immune complex deposition is thought to drive the pathogenesis of Libman-Sacks endocarditis. Consistent with this, antiphospholipid antibodies have been identified at the center of valvular lesions.[68] Several studies have found an association between antiphospholipid antibodies and the presence of valvular dysfunction. In particular, anti-cardiolipin antibodies have been identified in tissue sections of the affected valves.[68]

Other reported manifestations of valvular disease in SLE include valvulitis, aortic insufficiency, aortic stenosis, and mitral insufficiency. The mortality risk of surgical valve replacement is higher in patients with SLE and especially in patients taking immunosuppression.[69] Transcatheter valve replacement might be a safer option in some cases, although there are still limited data with regard transcatheter valve replacement in patients with SLE.[70]

SUMMARY

The heart is one of the most frequently affected organs in SLE. Any part of the heart can be affected, including the pericardium, myocardium, coronary arteries, valves, and the conduction system. In addition to pericarditis and myocarditis, a high inci-dence of CAD has become increasingly recognized as a cause of mortality, especially in older adult patients and those with long-standing SLE. Many unanswered questions remain in terms of understanding the pathogenesis of cardiac manifestations of SLE. It is not currently possible to predict the patients who are at greatest risk for the various types of cardiac involvement. However, with the rapid advancement of basic science and translational research approaches, it is now becoming easier to identify specific mutations associated with SLE. A better understanding of these genetic factors may eventually allow clinicians to categorize and predict the patients who are at risk for specific cardiac manifestations of SLE.

REFERENCES

1. Scott JS, Maddison PJ, Taylor PV, et al. Connective-tissue disease, antibodies to ribonucleoprotein, and congenital heart block. N Engl J Med 1983;309:209–12.
2. Lee LA. Transient autoimmunity related to maternal autoantibodies: neonatal lupus. Autoimmun Rev 2005;4:207–13.
3. Saleeb S, Copel J, Friedman D, et al. Comparison of treatment with fluorinated glucocorticoids to the natural history of autoantibody-associated congenital heart block: retrospective review of the research registry for neonatal lupus. Arthritis Rheum 1999;42:2335–45.
4. Buyon JP, Hiebert R, Copel J, et al. Autoimmune-associated congenital heart block: demographics, mortality, morbidity and recurrence rates obtained from a national neonatal lupus registry. J Am Coll Cardiol 1998;31:1658–66.
5. Jayaprasad N, Johnson F, Venugopal K. Congenital complete heart block and maternal connective tissue disease. Int J Cardiol 2006;112:153–8.
6. Friedman D, Rupel A, Buyon J. Epidemiology, etiology, detection, and treatment of autoantibody-associated congenital heart block in neonatal lupus. Curr Rheu-matol Rep 2007;9:101–8.
7. Lazzerini PE, Acampa M, Guideri F, et al. Prolongation of the corrected QT inter-val in adult patients with anti-Ro/SSA– positive connective tissue diseases. Arthritis Rheum 2004;50:1248–52.

8. Bourré-Tessier J, Clarke AE, Huynh T, et al. Prolonged corrected QT interval in anti-Ro/SSA–positive adults with systemic lupus erythematosus. Arthritis Care Res (Hoboken) 2011;63:1031-7.
9. Lazzerini PE, Capecchi PL, Guideri F, et al. Comparison of frequency of complex ventricular arrhythmias in patients with positive versus negative anti-Ro/SSA and connective tissue disease. Am J Cardiol 2007;100:1029-34.
10. Buyon J, Clancy R. Neonatal lupus: review of proposed pathogenesis and clinical data from the US-based Research Registry for Neonatal Lupus. Autoimmunity 2003;36:41-50.
11. Litsey SE, Noonan JA, O'Connor WN, et al. Maternal connective tissue disease and congenital heart block. N Engl J Med 1985;312:98-100.
12. Brucato A, Frassi M, Franceschini F, et al. Risk of congenital complete heart block in newborns of mothers with anti-Ro/SSA antibodies detected by counter-immunoelectrophoresis: a prospective study of 100 women. Arthritis Rheum 2001;44:1832-5.
13. Julkunen H, Eronen M. The rate of recurrence of isolated congenital heart block: a population-based study. Arthritis Rheum 2001;44:487-8.
14. Cooley H, Keech C, Melny B, et al. Monozygotic twins discordant for congenital complete heart block. Arthritis Rheum 1997;40:381-4.
15. Pisoni CN, Brucato A, Ruffatti A, et al. Failure of intravenous immunoglobulin to prevent congenital heart block: findings of a multicenter, prospective, observational study. Arthritis Rheum 2010;62:1147-52.
16. Hutter D, Silverman ED, Jaeggi ET. The benefits of transplacental treatment of isolated congenital complete heart block associated with maternal anti-Ro / SSA antibodies: a review. Scand J Immunol 2010;72:235-41.
17. Geggel R, Tucker L, Szer I. Postnatal progression from second- to third-degree heart block in neonatal lupus syndrome. J Pediatr 1988;113:1049-52.
18. Izmirly PM, Costedoat-Chalumeau N, Pisoni CN, et al. Maternal use of hydroxy-chloroquine is associated with a reduced risk of recurrent anti-SSA/Ro-antibody–associated cardiac manifestations of neonatal lupus. Circulation 2012; 126:76-82.
19. Moder KG, Miller TD, Tazelaar HD. Cardiac involvement in systemic lupus erythematosus. Mayo Clin Proc 1999;74:275-84.
20. Galve E, Candell-Riera J, Pigrau C, et al. Prevalence, morphologic types, and evolution of cardiac valvular disease in systemic lupus erythematosus. N Engl J Med 1988;319:817-23.
21. Starkey RH, Hahn BH. Rapid development of constrictive pericarditis in a patient with systemic lupus erythematosus. Chest 1973;63:448-50.
22. Jacobson E, Reza M. Constrictive pericarditis in systemic lupus erythematosus. Demonstration of immunoglobulins in the pericardium. Arthritis Rheum 1978;21: 972-4.
23. Cauduro SA, Moder KG, Tsang TS, et al. Clinical and echocardiographic characteristics of hemodynamically significant pericardial effusions in patients with systemic lupus erythematosus. Am J Cardiol 2003;92:1370-2.
24. Rosenbaum E, Krebs E, Cohen M, et al. The spectrum of clinical manifestations, outcome and treatment of pericardial tamponade in patients with systemic lupus erythematosus: a retrospective study and literature review. Lupus 2009;18:608-12.
25. Kahl L. The spectrum of pericardial tamponade in systemic lupus erythematosus. Report of ten patients. Arthritis Rheum 1992;35:1343-9.
26. Carroll N, Barrett J. Systemic lupus erythematosus presenting with cardiac tamponade. Br Heart J 1984;51:452-3.

27. Arabi MT, Malek EM, Fares MH, et al. Cardiac tamponade as the first manifestation of systemic lupus erythematosus in children. BMJ Case Rep 2012 [Epub ahead print].
28. Lindop R, Arentz G, Thurgood LA, et al. Pathogenicity and proteomic signatures of autoantibodies to Ro and La. Immunol Cell Biol 2012;90:304–9.
29. Quismorio FP Jr. Immune complexes in the pericardial fluid in systemic lupus erythematosus. Arch Intern Med 1980;140:112–4.
30. Suarez-Almazor M, Gonzalez-Lopez L, Gamez-Nava J, et al. Utilization and predictive value of laboratory tests in patients referred to rheumatologists by primary care physicians. J Rheumatol 1998;25:1980–5.
31. Imazio M, Spodick DH, Brucato A, et al. Controversial issues in the management of pericardial diseases. Circulation 2010;121:916–28.
32. Apte M, McGwin G, Vilá LM, et al, LUMINA Study Group. Associated factors and impact of myocarditis in patients with SLE from LUMINA, a multiethnic US cohort. Rheumatology 2008;47:362–7.
33. Doherty N, Siegel R. Cardiovascular manifestations of systemic lupus erythematosus. Am Heart J 1985;110:1257–65.
34. Jain D, Halushka MK. Cardiac pathology of systemic lupus erythematosus. J Clin Pathol 2009;62:584–92.
35. Saremi F, Ashikyan O, Saggar R, et al. Utility of cardiac MRI for diagnosis and post-treatment follow-up of lupus myocarditis. Int J Cardiovasc Imaging 2007;23:347–52.
36. Mavrogeni S, Bratis K, Markussis V, et al. The diagnostic role of cardiac magnetic resonance imaging in detecting myocardial inflammation in systemic lupus erythematosus. Differentiation from viral myocarditis. Lupus 2013;22:34–43.
37. Fairfax M, Osborn T, Williams G, et al. Endomyocardial biopsy in patients with systemic lupus erythematosus. J Rheumatol 1988;15:593–6.
38. Kavanagh D, Spitzer D, Kothari P, et al. New roles for the major human 3′- 5′ exonuclease TREX1 in human disease. Cell Cycle 2008;7:1718–25.
39. Lee-Kirsch MA, Gong M, Chowdhury D, et al. Mutations in the gene encoding the 3′-5′ DNA exonuclease TREX1 are associated with systemic lupus erythematosus. Nat Genet 2007;39:1065–7.
40. Morita M, Stamp G, Robins P, et al. Gene-targeted mice lacking the Trex1 (DNase III) 3′→5′ DNA exonuclease develop inflammatory myocarditis. Mol Cell Biol 2004;24:6719–27.
41. Rubin LA, Urowitz MB, Gladman DD. Mortality in systemic lupus erythematosus: the bimodal pattern revisited. QJM 1985;55:87–98.
42. Sumpter MD, Tatro LS, Stoecker WV, et al. Evidence for risk of cardiomyopathy with hydroxychloroquine. Lupus 2012;21:1594–6.
43. Vaccaro F, Caccavo D, Roumpedaki E, et al. Dilated cardiomyopathy due to thrombotic microangiopathy as the only manifestation of antiphospholipid syndrome: a case report. Int J Immunopathol Pharmacol 2008;21:237–41.
44. Abu-Shakra M, Urowitz M, Gladman D, et al. Mortality studies in systemic lupus erythematosus. Results from a single center. I. Causes of death. J Rheumatol 1995;22:1259–64.
45. Ward MM. Premature morbidity from cardiovascular and cerebrovascular diseases in women with systemic lupus erythematosus. Arthritis Rheum 1999;42:338–46.
46. Heibel RH, O'Toole JD, Curtiss EI, et al. Coronary arteritis in systemic lupus erythematosus. Chest 1976;69:700–3.
47. Bonfiglio T, Botti R, Hagstrom J. Coronary arteritis, occlusion, and myocardial infarction due to lupus erythematosus. Am Heart J 1972;83:153–8.

48. Artenjak A, Lakota K, Frank M, et al. Antiphospholipid antibodies as non-traditional risk factors in atherosclerosis based cardiovascular diseases without overt autoimmunity. A critical updated review. Autoimmun Rev 2012;11:873–82.
49. Sherer Y, Gerli R, Gilburd B, et al. Thickened carotid artery intima-media in rheumatoid arthritis is associated with elevated anticardiolipin antibodies. Lupus 2007;16:259–64.
50. Ishikawa S, Segar WE, Gilbert EF, et al. Myocardial infarct in a child with systemic lupus erythematosus. Am J Dis Child 1978;132:696–9.
51. Manzi S, Meilahn EN, Rairie JE, et al. Age-specific incidence rates of myocardial infarction and angina in women with systemic lupus erythematosus: comparison with the Framingham study. Am J Epidemiol 1997;145:408–15.
52. Ridker PM, Rifai N, Rose L, et al. Comparison of C-reactive protein and low-density lipoprotein cholesterol levels in the prediction of first cardiovascular events. N Engl J Med 2002;347:1557–65.
53. Ettinger WH, Goldberg AP, Applebaum-Bowden D, et al. Dyslipoproteinemia in systemic lupus erythematosus: effect of corticosteroids. Am J Med 1987;83:503–8.
54. Petri M, Lakatta C, Magder L, et al. Effect of prednisone and hydroxychloroquine on coronary artery disease risk factors in systemic lupus erythematosus: a longitudinal data analysis. Am J Med 1994;96:254–9.
55. Karp I, Abrahamowicz M, Fortin PR, et al. Recent corticosteroid use and recent disease activity: independent determinants of coronary heart disease risk factors in systemic lupus erythematosus? Arthritis Care Res (Hoboken) 2008;59:169–75.
56. Salmon JE, Roman MJ. Subclinical atherosclerosis in rheumatoid arthritis and systemic lupus erythematosus. Am J Med 2008;121:S3–8.
57. Haque S, Bruce I. Therapy insight: systemic lupus erythematosus as a risk factor for cardiovascular disease. Nat Clin Pract Cardiovasc Med 2005;2:423–30.
58. Petri MA. Hydroxychloroquine use in the Baltimore Lupus Cohort: effects on lipids, glucose and thrombosis. Lupus 1996;5(Suppl 1):S16–22.
59. Petri MA, Kiani AN, Post W, et al. Lupus Atherosclerosis Prevention Study (LAPS). Ann Rheum Dis 2011;70:760–5.
60. Moreno PR, Lodder RA, Purushothaman KR, et al. Detection of lipid pool, thin fibrous cap, and inflammatory cells in human aortic atherosclerotic plaques by near- infrared spectroscopy. Circulation 2002;105:923–7.
61. Anania C, Gustafsson T, Hua X, et al. Increased prevalence of vulnerable atherosclerotic plaques and low levels of natural IgM antibodies against phosphorylcholine in patients with systemic lupus erythematosus. Arthritis Res Ther 2010;12:R214.
62. Boyle JJ. Association of coronary plaque rupture and atherosclerotic inflammation. J Pathol 1997;181:93–9.
63. Libman E, Sacks B. A hitherto undescribed form of valvular and mural endocarditis. Arch Intern Med 1924;33:701–7.
64. Moyssakis I, Tektonidou MG, Vasilliou VA, et al. Libman-Sacks endocarditis in systemic lupus erythematosus: prevalence, associations, and evolution. Am J Med 2007;120:636–42.
65. Roldan CA, Qualls CR, Sopko KS, et al. Transthoracic versus transesophageal echocardiography for detection of Libman-Sacks endocarditis: a randomized controlled study. J Rheumatol 2008;35:224–9.
66. Straaton K, Chatham W, Reveille J, et al. Clinically significant valvular heart disease in systemic lupus erythematosus. Am J Med 1988;85:645–50.

67. Paget S, Bulkley B, Grauer L, et al. Mitral valve disease of systemic lupus erythematosus. A cause of severe congestive heart failure reversed by valve replacement. Am J Med 1975;59:134–9.
68. Ziporen L, Goldberg I, Arad M, et al. Libman-Sacks endocarditis in the antiphospholipid syndrome: immunopathologic findings in deformed heart valves. Lupus 1996;5:196–205.
69. Ashikhmina EA, Schaff HV, Dearani JA, et al. Aortic valve replacement in the elderly: determinants of late outcome. Circulation 2011;124:1070–8.
70. Bert JS, Abdullah M, Dahle TG, et al. Transcatheter aortic valve replacement for advanced valvular disease in active SLE and APS. Lupus 2013;22:1046–9.

The Heart and Pediatric Rheumatology

Tiphanie Vogel, MD, PhD[a,b], Maleewan Kitcharoensakkul, MD[a,c],
Lampros Fotis, MD, PhD[a], Kevin Baszis, MD[a,*]

KEYWORDS

- Kawasaki disease • Acute rheumatic fever • Poststreptococcal reactive arthritis
- Systemic juvenile idiopathic arthritis • Juvenile dermatomyositis • Neonatal lupus
- Marfan syndrome

KEY POINTS

- Recent advances in Kawasaki disease have included attempts to define genes involved in its pathogenesis, including multiple genome-wide association studies.
- Although the pathogenesis of acute rheumatic fever is complex, there have been recent advances in the studies of rheumatic carditis, leading to a better understanding of the mechanism of the disease.
- Histologic evaluation of patients with neonatal lupus erythematosus has revealed fibrosis with collagen deposition and calcification of the atrioventricular node, but disease can also extend to the sinoatrial node and the bundle of His.
- In Marfan syndrome, the abnormality of the mitral valve includes redundant elongation of one or both valve leaflets, often accompanied by myxomatous thickening.
- Therapy for cardiac involvement in systemic juvenile idiopathic arthritis should involve treatment of the underlying disease and systemic inflammatory state, and typically includes nonsteroidal antiinflammatory drugs, corticosteroids, disease-modifying drugs, and biologic therapies targeting tumor necrosis factor-alpha, interleukin-1, and interleukin-6.

KAWASAKI DISEASE

First described in 1967, Kawasaki disease is a systemic vasculitis that is typically acute, self-limited, and without sequelae. However, 15% to 25% of untreated patients develop coronary artery aneurysms, which can lead to fatality by myocardial infarction

No disclosures for any author.
[a] Division of Rheumatology, Department of Pediatrics, Washington University School of Medicine, Box 8116, One Children's Place, St Louis, MO 63110, USA; [b] Division of Rheumatology, Department of Medicine, Washington University School of Medicine, 660 South Euclid Avenue, St Louis, MO 63110, USA; [c] Division of Allergy/Immunology, Department of Pediatrics, Washington University School of Medicine, One Children's Place, St Louis, MO 63110, USA
* Corresponding author.
E-mail address: baszis_k@kids.wustl.edu

Rheum Dis Clin N Am 40 (2014) 61–85
http://dx.doi.org/10.1016/j.rdc.2013.10.008
0889-857X/14/$ – see front matter © 2014 Elsevier Inc. All rights reserved.

rheumatic.theclinics.com

or sudden death, which occurs in 0.17% of US patients with Kawasaki disease.[1] If the coronary artery aneurysms do not regress or resolve, ischemic heart disease can develop because of coronary artery stenosis or thrombosis. As the incidence of acute rheumatic fever has declined, Kawasaki disease has become the primary cause of acquired heart disease for children in industrialized countries.[1] In 2006 it was estimated that Kawasaki disease cost $110 million dollars in the United States,[2] making it a considerable financial burden.

Diagnosis

The typical patient with Kawasaki disease is a boy (1.5–1.7 male to 1 female incidence in the United States), aged 1 to 4 years old (76% of US patients are less than 5 years of age), who is appears unwell and is irritable.[1,3] Kawasaki disease occurs most commonly in Japan, with an incidence of 217 per 100,000 children less than 5 years old.[2] In the United States, passive surveillance data suggest that about 19 per 100,000 children develop Kawasaki disease.[2] For unexplained reasons, the incidence has been increasing in Japan but has remained stable in the United States.[2]

There is no diagnostic test for Kawasaki disease, thus diagnosis is based on a collection of criteria (**Box 1**). These criteria are fever greater than 39°C for 5 or more days, and at least 4 of 5 specific clinical findings (conjunctivitis, cervical lymphadenopathy, changes to the extremities, rash, and erythema of the lips/oral mucosa), in the absence of another explanatory cause. The diagnosis can be made on day 4 of fever if 4 of the other 5 criteria are present. However, the criteria do not necessarily present concurrently, which can lead to delayed diagnosis.[1]

The conjunctivitis of Kawasaki disease is bilateral, nonexudative, and typically is not painful. The extremity changes can be acute, including edema and/or induration, or can be delayed up to 2 to 3 weeks, as in the case of desquamation of the skin, which typically begins under the fingernails and can progress to include the palms and soles. The rash is most commonly an erythematous, maculopapular exanthem and can be especially prominent in the perineal area, which may peel during the acute illness. Cervical lymphadenopathy greater than 1.5 cm, which is usually located in the anterior chain and unilateral, is the least common of the 5 criteria.[1] If a patient has exudative conjunctivitis, exudative pharyngitis, discrete intraoral lesions, a bullous or vesicular rash, or generalized lymphadenopathy, Kawasaki disease is less likely, and alternative causes should be pursued.[1]

There is no laboratory finding diagnostic of Kawasaki disease or included in the criteria, but several findings can be used to support the diagnosis. An increased erythrocyte sedimentation rate (ESR) is found in 60% of patients,[4] increased C-reactive protein (CRP) in 80%,[4] neutrophil-predominant leukocytosis in 50%,[4] and sterile

---

Box 1
Criteria for the diagnosis of Kawasaki disease

Fever greater than 39°C for 5 days and 4 of the following 5 clinical findings:

Bilateral, nonexudative conjunctivitis

Changes to the extremities

Rash

Erythema of the lips/oral mucosa

Cervical lymphadenopathy greater than 1.5 cm

pyuria (>10 white blood cells per high-powered field) in 33%.[1] Hyponatremia, increased transaminases (especially alanine aminotransferase [ALT]), dyslipidemia, hypoalbuminemia, anemia, and thrombocytosis (although usually not present until after day 7 of illness) are also frequent findings.[1] Other common clinical findings include arthritis, hydrops of the gallbladder in 15% of patients,[1] uveitis, and aseptic meningitis in 50% of patients with Kawasaki disease.[1]

The American Heart Association criteria for the diagnosis of Kawasaki disease help prevent overdiagnosis but can fail to identify all patients with the condition.[1] Patients with fever for more than 5 days but only 2 or 3 of the clinical criteria can be diagnosed with incomplete Kawasaki disease, which occurs in up to 15% to 20% of patients.[4] Incomplete presentations are more common in infants less than 6 months of age or in older children. It has been advised that febrile infants without a fever source should have an echocardiogram after 7 days of fever to evaluate for Kawasaki disease to avoid missing an incomplete presentation.[1] In most cases, Kawasaki disease is an isolated occurrence, but it can recur in about 3% of patients.[1]

Multiple investigators have searched for a biomarker for use in the diagnosis of Kawasaki disease, particularly for cases that do not fulfill all the criteria, to help identify incomplete presentations. Several candidate proteins have been increased in the blood of patients with Kawasaki disease, including brain natriuretic peptide, S100 isoform A12, and meprin A, but none of these are in clinical use at this time.[4,5]

Atypical presentations of Kawasaki disease can include the presence of myocarditis, pericarditis, or Kawasaki disease shock syndrome.[4,6] Myocarditis can lead to ventricular dysfunction, valvular regurgitation from valvulitis, and conduction abnormalities.[4] Kawasaki shock syndrome occurs in about 7% of cases, more commonly in older children, and can manifest with hypotension, hemodynamic instability, or more severe coronary artery involvement, and is often resistant to first-line treatment.[6]

Coronary involvement in Kawasaki disease is evaluated at the time of diagnosis using echocardiography. Aneurysms are defined either by a coronary artery z score of greater than or equal to 2.5 (z scores reflect the intraluminal diameter relative to the patient's body surface area) in the left anterior descending (LAD) artery or right coronary artery (RCA) or by any 3 of the following echocardiographic criteria: z score of 2 to 2.4, perivascular brightness, lack of vessel tapering, decreased left ventricular function, mitral regurgitation, or pericardial effusion.[1] Aneurysms are most common in the proximal LAD and proximal RCA, followed by the left main coronary artery and left circumflex artery.[1]

The incidence of coronary artery aneurysms in treated patients in the United States is approximately 4%, with a lower incidence of 1% historically reported in Japanese patients.[2] However, recent data, suggest that Japanese patients are at higher risk of coronary artery aneurysms,[7] as are younger patients, male patients, those patients treated more than 10 days after the onset of illness, and those patients refractory to initial treatment.[1] Patients with incomplete Kawasaki disease also seem to be at higher risk for the development of aneurysms.[8] All coronary artery aneurysms are not detected at the time of diagnosis, and follow-up echocardiography 6 to 8 weeks later is recommended for further evaluation. If no coronary dilatation is detected at that time, it is thought that the risk of future aneurysm development is so low that no further imaging is recommended.[1]

Pathophysiology

Histologic analysis of vessels affected by inflammation in Kawasaki disease has been performed. Affected vessels first are noted to have edema of the media, with the internal elastic lamina remaining intact. At 7 to 9 days of illness, neutrophilic infiltration is noted, but this transitions to infiltration of lymphocytes, predominantly CD8+ T cells and immunoglobulin (Ig) A–secreting plasma cells, and the internal elastic lamina is destroyed. Fibroblast proliferation follows, leading to remodeling with fibrosis and scar formation.[1] The exact triggers of this process are unknown but remain under investigation.

Approximately 1% of patients with Kawasaki disease have a family history of the condition,[1] suggesting at least a partial genetic basis for the disease. This idea is supported by the finding that Asian populations retain the increased incidence of Kawasaki disease even after immigration to lower-incidence countries. For instance, the Japanese-American population of the state of Hawaii has an incidence of Kawasaki disease nearly equal to that found in Japan (210 per 100,000 children less than 5 years old).[2] However, there is only a 13% concordance rate for the development of Kawasaki disease among twins, suggesting that there is a strong environmental component as well.

Recent advances in Kawasaki disease have included attempts to define genes involved in the pathogenesis, including multiple genome-wide association studies. These efforts have identified several biologically plausible genes based on the known role of their protein products in the immune system. A polymorphism in CD40 ligand, a molecule involved in the costimulation of T cells, has been identified as a possible contributor in Japanese patients.[9] In both Japanese patients and patients of European ancestry, polymorphisms have been found in caspase-3, an enzyme fundamental to apoptosis, as well as in the high-affinity IgG receptor.[9] Whether these findings will be proved to be clinically relevant in Kawasaki disease remains to be determined.

The most promising genetic finding thus far has been the identification of a polymorphism in the gene for inositol 1,4,5-triphosphate kinase-C (ITPKC), a negative regulator of calcium signaling in activated T cells. This polymorphism has been associated with susceptibility to the development of Kawasaki disease in Japanese patients and to the development of coronary artery aneurysms in both Japanese and US patients.[10] This finding is particularly interesting because therapeutic agents that target calcium signaling pathways in T cells already exist, used most often for the prevention of solid organ transplant rejection, and are already being considered for use in Kawasaki disease (management of Kawasaki disease is discussed later). Given the increasing ease of this method and its power to identify single genes responsible for disease, the future of genetic studies in Kawasaki disease will likely be targeted at whole-exome sequencing of patients with particularly severe clinical manifestations, such as multiple giant coronary artery aneurysms.[9]

Although the cause of Kawasaki disease is unclear, it is thought that genetic influences are only part of the picture. An infectious source has long been speculated and aggressively sought out but has not been discovered. There are several features of Kawasaki disease that support an infectious trigger in the setting of a genetically predisposed patient. However, a primarily autoimmune origin is generally thought to be less likely, because of the self-limited nature of most cases and the lack of recurrence.[10] Seasonal variation to the incidence of Kawasaki disease supports an infectious source, although that seasonality is different in different locations: winter and early spring in the United States versus winter and midsummer in Japan.[2] There are also clear episodes of epidemics of the disease, such as occurred in Japan in 1979, 1982, and 1986, and in Finland in 1982.[2]

Antibodies synthesized using the immunoglobulin sequences of IgA plasma cells from patients with Kawasaki disease have recently been used to stain tissue sections from patients with Kawasaki disease and from control patients. These antibodies stained tissue from patients with Kawasaki disease but not from the controls. The staining was located in intracytoplasmic inclusion bodies, which contained a mixture of protein and RNA. It remains to be seen whether further investigation into this finding will lead to the identification of a previously unknown virus as a potential cause of Kawasaki disease.[10]

Management

The American Heart Association guidelines for treatment of Kawasaki disease address both the need to acutely decrease vessel inflammation as well as prevention of thrombosis in the presence of coronary artery aneurysms, because dilation results in areas of stasis of blood flow. The mainstays of Kawasaki treatment are intravenous immunoglobulin (IVIG) and aspirin. Treatment in a patient who fulfills criteria for Kawasaki disease should not be delayed if an echocardiogram cannot immediately be performed.[1]

In the United States, treatment using 2 g/kg of IVIG as a single infusion over 10 to 12 hours is recommended before day 10 of illness, and its use is supported by randomized, controlled evidence.[1,6] Treatment before day 5 has not been shown to be of benefit and may lead to increased need for retreatment. In contrast, if a patient presents after 10 days, but has continuing signs of inflammation (such as persistent fever), that patient should still be treated. With IVIG treatment, the incidence of coronary artery aneurysms is decreased from between 20% and 25% to between 1% and 4%. Treatment with IVIG also decreases fever duration and markers of inflammation.[11] The mechanism by which IVIG works is not clear, but many theories have been postulated, including IVIG neutralization of microbial toxins, impairment of an overabundant immune response (such as neutralizing host cytokines), decrease of endothelial activation, enhancement of T regulatory cell activity, or interference with production of antibody by B cells.[4,11]

Although aspirin is also recommended in the acute management of Kawasaki disease, there is no evidence that it improves outcomes; it has not been shown to decrease the incidence of coronary artery aneurysms.[4] In the United States, it is typically given at high dosage (80–100 mg/kg/d divided into 4 doses) until the patient has been afebrile for 48 hours. The dosage is then decreased to 3 to 5 mg/kg/d and continued until the patient has the recommended 6-week to 8-week follow-up echocardiogram. The aspirin is discontinued at that time if there is no evidence of coronary involvement.[1] If coronary artery aneurysms are present, the patient remains on low-dose aspirin until resolution of the aneurysms can be documented, or permanently if coronary changes persist. If the aneurysms are giant (>8 mm in diameter), anticoagulation with warfarin is also indicated. Low-molecular-weight heparin can also be used.[1]

Despite it being a systemic vasculitis, systemic corticosteroid treatment of Kawasaki is not part of the standard initial management strategy. In the past, this was likely because of an early report (before IVIG was used for Kawasaki disease) suggesting that steroid use worsened coronary artery outcomes, which was based on unrandomized data and has not been supported by subsequent evidence.[11] Recent randomized, controlled data in the United States showed no additional benefit from the addition of steroids to the standard initial management of Kawasaki disease. However, post hoc analysis of these data indicated that, in patients who failed initial management, coronary artery outcomes were better in patients who had received systemic corticosteroids.[12] Recent studies from Japan have also suggested that patients at high risk of developing coronary artery aneurysms benefited from use of steroids in initial management.[11] Efforts are now focused on developing ways to accurately identify high-risk patients who may benefit from initial use of adjunctive corticosteroids.[12] No algorithms are currently available for this.

Approximately 10% to 15% of patients with Kawasaki disease have persistent fever despite treatment with IVIG.[1] These patients are more likely to be male, have increased CRP or ALT, be thrombocytopenic, have recurrent Kawasaki disease, or have received initial IVIG treatment before day 5 of illness. Patients with IVIG-refractory disease are at increased risk of developing coronary artery aneurysms.[1] In IVIG-refractory patients, the American Heart Association guidelines for treatment of Kawasaki disease recommend the use of a second dose of IVIG 2 g/kg. This second dose is effective at terminating fever in 80% of refractory patients.[11]

Unlike initial management, decisions on how to treat patients with Kawasaki disease that has not responded to 2 doses of IVIG is guided mainly by case reports and small series. The most frequently used options include use of systemic corticosteroids or the use of tumor necrosis factor-alpha (TNF-α) inhibitors, mainly infliximab or etanercept. The guidelines from the American Heart Association, based on expert opinion, recommend the use of intravenous (IV) methylprednisolone 30 mg/kg daily for 1 to 3 days if there is disease persistence beyond the second dose of IVIG.[1]

Use of TNF-α inhibitors is based on the finding of increased TNF in the serum of patients with Kawasaki disease, and on mouse models of Kawasaki disease showing that blockade of TNF or absence of TNF signaling decreases coronary artery inflammation.[6] Infliximab has been shown to be safe when used in Kawasaki disease as second-line treatment in patients unresponsive to a first dose of IVIG, but this study was not powered to show whether there was a difference between treatment groups.[12] A randomized, controlled trial of the use of infliximab as an adjunct to standard initial treatment is currently underway in the United States. A pilot study of etanercept has shown it to be well tolerated when used with initial IVIG treatment, and a randomized, controlled trial has been proposed to further investigate its potential to decrease IVIG-resistant disease.[12]

Other agents have been used for IVIG-refractory Kawasaki disease and reported in case reports. Based on the recent findings (discussed earlier) of polymorphisms in the ITPKC gene associated with the development of coronary artery aneurysms in Kawasaki disease, use of cyclosporine for treatment-refractory disease has been reported. Cyclosporine interferes with calcium signaling in T cells, the pathway involving ITPKC. In 9 of 9 reported IVIG-refractory patients receiving cyclosporine, fever and markers of inflammation were decreased after cyclosporine use.[11]

Prognosis

Algorithms for identifying patients at high risk for the development of coronary aneurysms ideally will be created and validated, and more intensive treatments can be directed to further reduce the incidence of cardiac sequelae of Kawasaki disease. At this time, patients who develop aneurysms are at risk for persistence of the aneurysms and the development of artery stenosis or thrombosis. However, half of aneurysms show angiographic evidence of resolution within 1 to 2 years of diagnosis.[4] Aneurysms more likely to regress are those that are smaller, in patients less than 1 year of age, fusiform (vs saccular), and in a distal artery location.[1] Giant aneurysms (those >8 mm) are unlikely to regress and can lead to stenosis or occlusion (74%), myocardial infarction (31%), and/or the need for coronary artery bypass grafting (19%).[2]

Cardiology follow-up for patients with Kawasaki disease is determined by several factors. Patients with no aneurysms or regression of aneurysms by the 6-week to 8-week follow-up echocardiogram have no specific recommendation for follow-up aside from standard counseling regarding cardiac health. Patients with persistent aneurysms should be followed serially with cardiology evaluation and counseling, electrocardiogram, echocardiography, and stress testing, at intervals based on the degree of coronary artery dilatation, with activity restrictions based on the results of stress testing. Initial angiography within 6 to 12 months is recommended for patients with giant aneurysms and in other patients if ischemia is noted on stress testing.[1] Evaluation using MRI, CT, or intraluminal ultrasound is still investigational.[4]

Angioplasty or coronary artery stenting by interventional cardiology has only been performed in a small population of patients with Kawasaki disease. Good outcomes have been reported, especially if done within the first 2 years after disease onset, although there is a high rate of recurrence of stenosis.[4] Coronary artery bypass grafting is sometimes required in patients with giant aneurysms and persistent ischemia, with reported outcomes of 95% survival at 25 years and 60% cardiac event–free survival at 25 years.[4] Cardiac transplant is reserved only for a select set of patients with irreversible cardiac dysfunction and lesions that cannot be addressed with interventional cardiology procedures or surgical bypass grafting.[1]

It was previously thought that patients with Kawasaki disease and coronary artery aneurysms that regress proceed to have a normal future cardiac risk. However, there is accumulating histologic and functional (vessel response to vasodilators) data that areas of previous aneurysm remain abnormal.[1] This finding has led to speculation that these patients have an increased future cardiac risk, in particular in the development of atherosclerotic lesions in these previously dilated areas. At this time, there is no evidence available to suggest that these patients require more specialized cardiac follow-up than the standard counseling on lifestyle modifications that are suggested for all adult patients, including advice regarding abstinence from tobacco use, healthy diet choices, regular aerobic exercise to avoid the development of obesity, as well as treatment of hypertension and dyslipidemia when necessary.[13] Future studies should include trials of statins in patients with Kawasaki disease who may be at risk of accelerated atherosclerosis.[13]

ACUTE RHEUMATIC FEVER

Acute rheumatic fever (ARF) is an immune-mediated disease that can follow untreated streptococcal pharyngitis, leading to inflammation of joints, heart, skin, or brain. ARF causes significant morbidity and mortality because of chronic damage to heart valves and rheumatic heart disease (RHD), and this remains a global burden of disease caused by group A streptococcal infection.[14] Although the pathogenesis of ARF is complex, there have been recent advances in the study of rheumatic carditis, leading to a better understanding of the mechanism of the disease. In contrast, there is a paucity of new data for the treatment of this disease.

Epidemiology

The prevalence of ARF varies with the geographic region, rural versus urban setting, socioeconomic conditions, and age group. Although the incidence and prevalence of ARF and RHD have been decreasing in developed countries since the early 1900s, they continue to be major causes of morbidity and mortality among young people in developing countries. In 2005, Carepetis and colleagues[15] estimated that 15.6 million to 19.6 million people worldwide have RHD, and at least 2.4 million people were children aged 5 to 14 years. They also estimated that at least 200,000 to 250,000 premature cardiovascular deaths are caused by RHD every year.

The highest incidence of ARF has been reported among the Aboriginals and Torres Strait islanders of Australia and the Maoris of New Zealand.[16] In 2000, Oen and colleagues[17] compared the incidence rate of ARF per 100,000 persons in each region. Incidence was low in industrialized nations (0.23–1.14), 15.2 among African American populations in Florida, 125 in Sri Lanka, 142 among Maori in New Zealand, 206 in Samoans in Hawaii, and up to 650 in Australian aboriginal groups. Although the incidence of ARF has decreased in all regions over the past 20 years, the reported prevalence of RHD is increasing in all regions except for Europe, which may be because of advances in medical and surgical treatments for RHD that have led to increased survival in these patients,[14] as well as increased screening for RHD by echocardiography in countries with high disease prevalence. The incidence of RHD does not necessarily correspond with that of ARF, and the explanation is likely multifactorial.[18] In 2005, the incidence of RHD was highest in Africa, the Pacific, and south-central Asia.[15]

ARF and RHD are more common in rural than urban populations.[19] ARF is also more common in low socioeconomic areas,[20,21] which could be secondary to limited access to medical care, poor medical attention, hygiene, malnutrition, poor adherence to prophylaxis, and increased household crowding leading to increased streptococcal exposure. Most studies have shown that men and women are equally affected; however, from a recent worldwide epidemiologic study, there is a slight male predominance.[14]

The initial attack of ARF is most common just before adolescence, ranging from 5 to 14 years old, less common near the end of the second decade, and rare in adults older than age 35 years.[16] ARF can also first occur in children younger than 5 years, representing approximately 5% to 10% of patients with ARF.[22–24] RHD usually results from the cumulative damage of recurrent episodes of ARF, thus the prevalence of RHD increases with age, peaking in adults aged 25 to 34 years, reflecting ARF activity in previous decades.[16]

Pathogenesis of Carditis in ARF

Streptococcus pyogenes, or group A beta-hemolytic streptococci (GAS), have long been known to be associated with the development of ARF. This knowledge is supported by the observations that outbreaks of ARF have followed outbreaks of pharyngitis and that increasing antistreptococcal antibodies are seen in patients with ARF.[25] Because GAS possess antigens and superantigens that can stimulate B and T cells to respond to self-proteins, a hypothesis of molecular mimicry between bacterial antigens (M protein[16,26] and carbohydrate antigen[16]) and cardiac proteins, particularly alpha-helical proteins such as myosin, laminin, and vimentin, on host tissues has been proposed.[27,28] The M protein is a major virulence factor for GAS, and initial observations showed that strains with certain serotypes of M protein were particularly associated with outbreak of ARF, giving rise to the hypothesis of so-called rheumatogenic strains of GAS.[29] However, with the advances of immunologic studies, the antibodies that target heart valves in humans are now thought to perhaps not target the M protein, but rather the carbohydrate antigen on certain streptococcal strains.[30] Studies by Adderson and colleagues[32] of antistreptococcal/antiheart monoclonal antibodies from rheumatic carditis have revealed that cardiac myosin and N-acetyl-B-D-glucosamine (NABG), the dominant epitope of the group A carbohydrate antigen, are the cross-reactive antigens involved in antibody deposition on valves.[31,32] However, myosin is present in myocardium but not in valve tissues, which are the major site affected by ARF. A subsequent study of mice immunized with streptococcal pyrogenic exotoxin B showed that the mice developed autoantibodies that can cross react with NABG and endothelial cells, again supporting the molecular mimicry hypothesis and possibly explaining the valvulitis in patients with RHD.[33] In addition, a recent study showed the presence of anti–endothelial cell antibodies (AECA) in 40% of Yemeni patients with RHD.[34] A subsequent study by this group showed that vimentin is the potential autoantigen for AECA. They were able to show cross reactivity of purified antivimentin antibodies with heat shock protein-70 and streptopain strepto-coccal proteins, and these antibodies were able to activate microvascular cardiac endothelium by amplifying the inflammatory response in RHD.[35]

Given that pathologic and immunologic findings suggest that the primary site of rheumatic fever–related damage is the subendothelial collagen matrix, another hypothesis of ARF has recently emerged. Studies by Dinkla and colleagues suggest that M protein of rheumatogenic streptococcal strains binds and forms a complex with the CB3 region in human collagen type IV in subendothelial basement mem-branes,[36,37] and that this immune complex might initiate an autoantibody response to the collagen as seen in patients with Goodpasture or Alport syndromes.[30] More-over, these antibodies do not cross react with M proteins, and this hypothesis argues against the molecular mimicry concept. Further studies are ongoing to test this hypothesis.

Host susceptibility that is genetically determined has also been presumed to play a role in the pathogenesis of ARF, because of the difference of its prevalence in each geographic region, increased risk of RHD in certain populations, the tendency for out-breaks to occur within families,[38] and the strong association with the monozygosity and concordance rate of ARF.[39] With advances in genetic studies, different human leuko-cyte antigen (HLA) class II antigen associations have been observed in several popula-tions.[40] Several studies have reported an association of ARF with various genetic polymorphisms involved in regulation of both innate and adaptive immunity, including mannose-binding lectin, toll-like receptor-2 and ficolin-2, interleukin (IL)-1 receptor antagonist, TNF-α, transforming growth factor beta (TGF-β), cytotoxic T-lymphocyte antigen 4 (CTLA-4), IL-6, IL-10, and angiotensin-converting enzyme (ACE).[40–42]

Based on the molecular mimicry hypothesis, following a streptococcal infection, the susceptible host develops cross-reactive autoantibodies against group A strepto-coccal carbohydrate antigen, cardiac myosin in the myocardium, and endothelial cells of the valves. The valves become inflamed with expression of vascular cell adhesion molecule-1. After this event, CD4+ and CD8+ T cells infiltrate through the endothe-lium/endocardium into the valve. The valve becomes scarred with eventual neovascu-larization and progressive, chronic valvular disease.[31] In the past, ARF was thought to occur only following streptococcal pharyngitis, not impetigo and skin infections. How-ever, there is some epidemiologic evidence to suggest that skin strains of GAS may play a role in the pathogenesis of ARF. Further studies need to be performed to prove direct causation of ARF after skin infection.[18]

Diagnosis of ARF

The clinical manifestations of ARF occur 2 to 6 weeks after streptococcal pharyngitis. The diagnostic criteria for ARF were first developed by Jones[43] in 1944 and have been revised over the years,[44–46] with the most recent revision in 1992.[47] The criteria are divided into major and minor criteria (**Table 1**). The diagnosis of ARF is made by the presence of 2 major criteria or of 1 major and 2 minor criteria, plus evidence of a pre-ceding streptococcal infection. Clinicians should be aware that the Jones criteria were developed for, and are applicable only to, initial attacks of ARF.[47] A diagnosis of ARF can be made without fulfilling criteria if any of these are present: chorea, indolent car-ditis, or recurrent episodes of ARF. Patients with chorea and indolent carditis are not required to have evidence of streptococcal infection, because these can be late man-ifestations of ARF.[47] Diagnosis of recurrent episodes of ARF can be based on only minor manifestations and evidence of recent streptococcal infection in patients with preexisting RHD, because patients with RHD have a high risk of carditis in recurrent ARF.[18,48] In developing countries, especially among high-incident indigenous

Table 1
1992 updated Jones criteria for the diagnosis of a first episode of ARF

Major Criteria	Minor Criteria
Polyarthritis	• Fever
Carditis	• Arthralgias
Erythema marginatum	• Elevated acute phase reactants
Subcutaneous nodules	• PR interval prolongation
Chorea	

Evidence of streptococcal infection including increased or increasing streptococcal antibody titer or positive group A streptococcal throat culture or rapid streptococcal antigen test.

Adapted from Guidelines for the diagnosis of rheumatic fever. Jones criteria, 1992 update. Special Writing Group of the Committee on Rheumatic Fever, Endocarditis, and Kawasaki Disease of the Council on Cardiovascular Disease in the Young of the American Heart Association. JAMA 1992;268(15):2069–73.

populations, epidemiologists have noted that strict application of the updated Jones criteria may result in underdiagnosis of ARF.[49]

With the first episode of ARF, arthritis is the most common manifestation (60%–75%), carditis is the second most common manifestation (40%–60%), followed by chorea (6%–15%), erythema marginatum (4%–11%), and subcutaneous nodules (5%–7%).[24,48,50] In certain populations, carditis is the most common manifestation and is reported to occur in 79% of cases in Fiji and Australia.[51] In addition, up to 88% of patients with chorea had abnormal echocardiographic findings.[52] Regarding the minor criteria, fever (>37.5°C) was found in 30% to 40%, arthralgia in 80%, increased ESR and CRP in 70% to 80%, and prolonged PR interval in 30% to 40% of patients with ARF.[53,54]

Cardiac Manifestations of ARF

Carditis is the most severe clinical feature of ARF because of its long-term sequelae from chronic damage to cardiac valves. Patients with ARF who develop carditis usually present with new heart murmurs, tachycardia, pericarditis, or congestive heart failure.[54] Up to one-third of patients can present with congestive heart failure at diagnosis.[53] Although the revision of the Jones criteria in 1992 emphasized that rheumatic carditis is almost always associated with a murmur of valvulitis, and patients with isolated myocarditis and/or pericarditis should be diagnosed with ARF with great caution,[47] ARF typically causes pancarditis.[30] All 4 heart valves can be involved, but there is a marked predominance of mitral valve (MV) involvement; the cause of this is unclear, because all heart valves develop from the same tissue.[14] ARF also affects the aortic, tricuspid, and pulmonic valves, in decreasing order.[19,24] Patients who recover from the initial rheumatic carditis are likely to have permanent valve damage, and over time the affected valves can became stenotic and/or regurgitant.[14] Given that silent or subclinical carditis was frequently reported in children presenting with ARF in endemic countries, and studies showed that Doppler echocardiography is more sensitive in detecting carditis than auscultation, echocardiography became an important tool and the most reliable noninvasive technique for the diagnosis of carditis.[55–57] Echocardiography is also helpful for determining the extent of disease. In patients with carditis at presentation, 30% to 70% may develop persistence of valvular abnormalities at 5 years; the frequency depends on the studied populations and adherence to secondary prophylaxis.[24,52,54,58] Risk factors for development of RHD include the severity of carditis at the first attack,[54] the number of valves involved at the first attack,[54] and the recurrent attack rate.[16,59] RHD developed in only 6% of patients who had no carditis with the initial attack.[58] All patients who became symptom-free at 1 year after diagnosis had only single valve involvement and mild to moderate carditis.[54]

Recurrent ARF occurs in approximately 8% of patients.[60] Based on a prospective study in Pakistan, carditis was more frequent in patients who had recurrent ARF (96% vs 60% with first episode), and patients with recurrent ARF had a higher frequency of moderate-severe carditis compared with patients who had ARF for the first time.[48] Because only 20% of patients with recurrent ARF had a history of sore throat, it is important to have a high index of suspicion in these patients.[48]

In addition, children younger than 5 years old with ARF were more likely to present with moderate to severe carditis.[22] This group of younger patients also can develop clinical RHD, which occurred in approximately 55% of those who initially had carditis.[22]

Treatment of Carditis

There is a paucity of recent data on treatment of ARF; most prior studies were not done in a randomized controlled fashion; and most studies were done in adults, whereas the onset of disease commonly occurs in older children and teenagers. The treatment of ARF is divided into 3 main categories: (1) heart failure management, (2) treatment with antiinflammatory agents, and (3) eradication of streptococcal infection.

Antiinflammatory agents can shorten the acute phase of ARF and improve symptoms of arthritis. Aspirin continues to be the mainstay of treatment of ARF and is typically given in the early phase at 80 to 100 mg/kg/d divided into 4 doses. However, naproxen was also shown to be as effective as aspirin, with fewer side effects.[61] It is recommended to continue aspirin for 4 to 6 weeks, until the clinical symptoms of ARF resolve, or until the normalization of inflammatory markers.[62] Some experts recommend the use of corticosteroids in treatment of severe carditis (ie, carditis with heart failure). However, this is not based on evidence that steroids reduce the risk of developing valvular lesions in this group of patients.[18] A retrospective study compared the long-term outcome of 118 patients with severe rheumatic carditis in Brazil. Patients with carditis received either intravenous methylprednisolone (30 mg/kg/d up to 3 courses per week for 2–5 courses) or oral prednisolone (2 mg/kg/d for 3 to 4 weeks followed by tapering), and there was no difference in the rate of severe valve regurgitation during the mean follow-up period of 7.7 years.[63] From a meta-analysis by Cilliers and colleagues,[64] there was no significant difference in the risk of cardiac disease at or after 1 year between corticosteroid-treated and aspirin-treated groups. IVIG has been used in a randomized controlled trial for patients with ARF; however, it did not alter the clinical course or lead to reduction in echocardiographic evidence of acute valvular heart disease or chronic damage 1 year later.[65] Because there are no treatments during the acute phase of carditis that have been shown to affect the outcome, it is important to emphasize the importance of good adherence to secondary prophylaxis. Once patients develop RHD, treatment is complex, including medications for heart failure, anticoagulation, cardiothoracic surgery, and/or interventional procedures.

Regarding eradication of streptococcal colonization/infection, although most patients with ARF no longer have active streptococcal infection, most experts recommend antibiotic therapy to eradicate any residual infection in the pharynx, even if throat cultures are negative. Intramuscular benzathine penicillin G and oral penicillin V are recommended for treatment of GAS.[66] The dose of benzathine penicillin G is 600,000 units for patients less than or equal to 27 kg and 1.2 million units for patients more than 27 kg, given intramuscularly for 1 dose. The dosage for oral penicillin V is 250 mg 2 to 3 times daily for patients less than or equal to 27 kg and 500 mg 2 to 3 times daily for patients more than 27 kg, for 10 days.[66] If patients are allergic to penicillin, acceptable alternatives include narrow-spectrum cephalosporins (cephalexin, cefadroxil), clindamycin, azithromycin, or clarithromycin. Once patients complete the treatment course for streptococcal infection, it is important to continue secondary prophylaxis to prevent recurrent attacks of ARF.

Prevention

Primary prophylaxis, including the timely treatment of streptococcal pharyngitis, has been shown to prevent ARF. The current focus of global efforts on prevention of RHD is on secondary prophylaxis (regular administration of penicillin to prevent recurrent ARF).[18] There have been attempts to use echocardiographic screening in countries with high prevalence of ARF, with the goal of detecting RHD in its early stages. Secondary prophylaxis has been shown to lead to regression of existing heart valve lesions and to reduce RHD mortality.

Similar to the antibiotics for primary GAS treatment, the agents of choice for secondary prophylaxis include benzathine penicillin G and penicillin V. If patients are allergic to penicillin, sulfadiazine can be used as an alternative. If patients are also allergic to sulfadiazine or do not tolerate the medication, they can use macrolides; however, there are no standard doses for this indication.[66]

The duration of prophylaxis depends on the severity of the lesion and the age of the patient. Based on the guidelines endorsed by the American Academy of Pediatrics in 2009, patients without carditis should continue on prophylaxis until 5 years after diagnosis of ARF or 21 years of age, whichever is longer. Patients with initial carditis without residual RHD should remain on prophylaxis until 10 years after diagnosis of ARF or 21 years of age, whichever is longer. Patients with ARF, carditis, and persistent valvular disease should continue prophylaxis for 10 years after diagnosis, until 40 years of age, or sometimes for life.[66] The recurrence rate of ARF is associated with compliancy with secondary prophylaxis.[58] In all situations, the decision to discontinue prophylaxis or to reinstate it should be made after discussion with the patient of the potential risks and benefits and careful consideration of the epidemiologic risk factors.[66]

POSTSTREPTOCOCCAL REACTIVE ARTHRITIS

Poststreptococcal reactive arthritis (PSRA) is another form of arthritis caused by GAS and is a common nonsuppurative complication following streptococcal infection. This term was first used in 1959 by Crea and Mortimer[67] to describe patients who had arthritis after an episode of GAS pharyngitis but lacked major criteria of ARF. Because the pathogenesis of PSRA and ARF are not completely understood, it is unclear whether PSRA is the same disease as ARF with a different spectrum or if they are distinct entities. In contrast with ARF occurring only after GAS infections, PSRA can follow groups A, C, or G streptococcal infection. Most cases of PSRA have been reported from the United States and western Europe; the incidence and prevalence rates are uncertain.[68] Based on a population-based study performed in Norway, PSRA accounts for 10% of all arthritis in children less than 16 years old.[69]

Clinical Presentation

The age of presentation for PSRA is bimodal, with a peak at the ages 8 to 14 years and another peak at 21 to 37 years of age.[70] Both genders are equally affected in all age groups.[62] Although patients with both ARF and PSRA can present with fever, arthritis, and increased inflammatory markers, there are disparities between their clinical presentations. The latency period between streptococcal infection and PSRA is shorter than ARF, being 7 to 10 days in PSRA versus 3 to 6 weeks in ARF. The pattern of polyarthritis in PSRA can be asymmetric or symmetric; however, it usually occurs in an additive and prolonged manner, rather than polyarticular and migratory as in ARF. PSRA does not promptly respond to aspirin or nonsteroidal antiinflammatory agents, in contrast with the good response in ARF. The mean duration of arthritis in PSRA is ~2 months and can be recurrent, whereas the arthritis in ARF usually peaks in the first week and resolves in less than 3 weeks.[68]

Carditis has been reported in PSRA,[71,72] but the data are conflicting, and the incidence is unknown. From an unselected cohort of 75 adult patients with PSRA who did not receive antibiotic prophylaxis and were followed prospectively for a mean duration of 8.9 years, there was no increased risk of valvular heart disease in patients compared with controls.[73] However, a retrospective study of 40 children with PSRA in the United States showed that 18% of patients had abnormal echocardiographic findings at follow-up visits, despite receiving antibiotic prophylaxis for a mean duration of 22 months. Most patients developed cardiac findings early in the disease course; there were only 2 patients who developed findings after 12 months of follow-up.[74] Another study of children in the United States reported outcomes of 12 children diagnosed with PSRA. None had carditis at diagnosis, but 1 patient developed classic ARF with valvulitis 18 months after the initial episode of PSRA.[75] The other features of ARF, including chorea, erythema marginatum, and subcutaneous nodules, have not been reported in PSRA. However, other skin lesions, including erythema nodosum, erythema multiforme, scarlatiniform, urticarial, or nonspecific rashes, have been observed in PSRA.[68] Tendinitis has been infrequently reported in PSRA. There is 1 report of tendinitis or enthesitis in 20% of 26 Arab/Asian patients with PSRA.[71]

There are no standardized criteria for the diagnosis of PSRA. Ayoub and colleagues[76] proposed a set of diagnostic criteria in 1997; however, these have not been systematically validated in populations. In general, the diagnosis of PSRA is based on arthritis, evidence of streptococcal infection (group A, C, or G), and lack of other Jones criteria.

The treatment of PSRA consists of symptomatic relief of arthritis and eradication of streptococcal infection. Based on the American Heart Association guideline in 2009, once a patient completes initial treatment with benzathine penicillin or penicillin V, secondary prophylaxis should be continued for at least 1 year after diagnosis and then discontinued if there is no evidence of carditis at 1 year.[66]

NEONATAL LUPUS ERYTHEMATOSUS

Neonatal lupus erythematosus (NLE) is a rare disease, caused by maternal autoantibodies crossing the placenta. The most severe clinical presentation of NLE is cardiac arrhythmias, but cutaneous, hepatic, and hematologic involvement are frequently present.[77] The cutaneous lesions persist for an average of 15 to 17 weeks and then resolve with the clearance of maternal antibodies from the infants circulation. Hepatic manifestations may include transaminase increase, liver cholestasis, and hepatic failure. The most common hematologic manifestation is thrombocytopenia, with petechiae and purpura being the prominent signs.[78] This article focuses on the cardiac manifestations of NLE.

Of the cardiac abnormalities, the most common in NLE is congenital atrioventricular block (AVB), which most often is a third-degree block and is strongly associated with the transplacental passage of maternal IgG antibodies reacting with the 48-kD SS-B/La, 52-kD SS-A/Ro, and 60-kD SS-A/Ro. Second-degree block is observed less frequently, and first-degree block is also rare.[79]

Two hypotheses have been proposed to explain the mechanism of injury by maternal autoantibodies. The first suggests that the antibodies cross react with L-type calcium channels (LTCC), causing dysregulation of calcium homeostasis.[79] Supporting this theory is an experimental study using 2 strains of transgenic mice. Mice overexpressing the LTCC had reduced rate of conduction abnormalities when exposed to anti–SS-A/Ro and SS-B/La antibodies, whereas LTCC knockout mice had significantly worse electrocardiographic abnormalities.[80] The second hypothesis is the apoptotic theory, according to which the responsible antibodies bind myocytes that undergo apoptosis during physiologic remodeling.[79] This event activates the uro-kinase plasminogen activator/urokinase plasminogen activator receptor complex, leading to plasmin generation, and, at the same time, impairs the removal of apoptotic cells by healthy myocardial cells.[81] Plasmin cleaves beta-2 glycoprotein I, which has been found to have protective properties for the myocardium through preventing the binding of anti–SS-A/Ro to the apoptotic myocardial cells.[82] The binding of anti–SS-A/Ro to apoptotic cardiac myocytes triggers TGF-β activation, which promotes scarring of tissue.[83]

In a recent US-based cohort study of mothers positive for anti–SS-A/Ro and previous pregnancies affected by cardiac NLE, 79.1% of the infants had a third-degree block.[84] In the same study population, SS-B/La antibodies were present in 64.3% of pregnancies and anti–52-kDa Ro antibody in 90.8%.[84] Women positive for the implicated antibodies have a risk of 2% for bearing a child with cardiac NLE in their first pregnancies.[85] The recurrence risk in subsequent pregnancies increases 8-fold to 9-fold, reaching approximately 17%, whereas the estimated recurrence rate after having 2 children with cardiac NLE is 50%.[86] The mortality is 17.5%, with 30% of these in utero. Cumulative probability of survival in 10 years is 86%.[84] The case fatality ranges from 11% to 29%, whereas 63% to 93% of children receive pacemakers.[84]

Other electrophysiologic abnormalities reported in NLE in addition to AVB are prolonged QT interval, atrial and ventricular ectopy, atrial flutter, ventricular and junctional tachycardia, and transient or persistent sinus node dysfunction.[87,88] In the absence of AVB, isolated transient QT prolongation, resolving within the first year of life,[89] and sinus bradycardia have been reported,[85] although both findings were not confirmed by other larger studies.[90]

Endocardial fibroelastosis (EFE) is a rare complication involving both the endocardium and myocardium. It usually leads to end-stage heart failure and has been reported in children with antibody-mediated AVB.[91] It predominantly involves the left ventricle in the postnatal infant and predominantly the right ventricle in the fetus, but it can also involve the crux of the heart, chordal apparatus, papillary muscles, and atria.[87,91,92] Not all patients with AVB develop EFE, and there are also reported series of isolated antibody-mediated EFE, without the presence of AVB, suggesting that EFE may occur by a different mechanism.[92,93] Nonetheless, EFE is considered a significant risk factor for death in patients with AVB.[94] Late-onset dilated cardiomyopathy leading to congestive heart failure is a sequela of complete AVB, despite the early institution of cardiac pacing.[95] In addition, pericardial effusion has been reported in fetuses.[96]

Anatomic cardiovascular abnormalities in conjunction with autoimmune-mediated congenital AVB have frequently been reported,[97] and include patent ductus arteriosus, atrial and ventricular septal defects, and semilunar and atrioventricular valve abnormalities.[87] The cause of the anatomic abnormalities is uncertain, but a combination of inflammation, fibrosis, and hemodynamic changes may contribute to the evolution of these lesions.[87]

Histologic evaluation of patients with NLE has revealed fibrosis with collagen deposition and calcification of the atrioventricular node, but disease can also extend to the sinoatrial node and the bundle of His. Valvular damage, including fibrosis and calcification of the papillary muscles, has also been reported. Inflammatory infiltrate involving the endocardium, myocardium, and pericardium has been reported, consisted with EFE and not always affecting the conduction system.[98]

No guidelines exist for the time and frequency of screening for AVB, but it seems that the most vulnerable period is between 18 and 24 weeks of gestation. A prudent approach includes weekly echocardiograms starting at the 18th week of gestation until the 26th week and then every other week up to the 32nd week.

Dexamethasone and betamethasone (fluorinated steroids) have been instituted for the treatment and prevention of AVB.[99] Steroids are not recommended after third-degree block has been established, because the AVB is irreversible, unless there are other factors that may improve with steroids, including pericardial and pleural effusions, hydrops fetalis, or ascites.[96] The use of steroids when alternating second-degree to third-degree block is present is controversial, although some investigators recommend their use.[99] When the initial abnormal rhythm is first-degree or second-degree block, reversal may be observed after steroid treatment.[99,100] The prenatal administration of 400 mg/kg of IVIG has not been proved to be effective in the prevention of AVB and is not currently recommended.[101,102] Treatment of the mother with hydroxychloroquine during pregnancy may decrease the risk of cardiac NLE.[103,104] For other cardiac manifestations, the combination of prednisone and IVIG before and after birth was promising for the treatment of cardiomyopathy/EFE.[105]

JUVENILE DERMATOMYOSITIS

Juvenile dermatomyositis (JDM) is a chronic autoimmune multisystem vasculopathy presenting with inflammation of striated muscle, skin, and other organs. This article focuses on the cardiac involvement in JDM, a rare manifestation.[106]

In adult studies of patients with dermatomyositis/polymyositis, the incidence of cardiac involvement ranges from 9% to 72%. The most prominent manifestations are heart failure, conduction abnormalities, and left ventricular diastolic and systolic dysfunction, with cardiac manifestations being one of the common causes of death.[107]

In a cohort of 25 children with JDM, the incidence of cardiac involvement was 12%, with 2 patients presenting with a conduction abnormality and 1 with myocarditis.[108] In a Hungarian national registry of 44 patients with JDM, none were reported to have cardiac involvement.[109] A recent study comparing patients with JDM with healthy controls revealed that patients with JDM had diastolic dysfunction, as defined by the measurement of early diastolic transmitral flow/early diastolic tissue velocity. Left ventricular stiffness and slower left ventricular relaxation was present, presumably as the result of myocardial remodeling. Pathologic diastolic dysfunction was combined with electrocardiogram abnormalities. Pericarditis was also observed.[110] Systolic dysfunction, measured using the mitral annulus displacement, was studied in the same population. Systolic dysfunction was correlated with cumulative organ damage and disease duration. There was also a correlation between diastolic dysfunction and high disease activity in the skin in the first year but not with muscle disease.[111] A limitation of both studies was that the studied population was examined 16.8 years (range 2–38 years) after disease diagnosis. The onset of the disease was in childhood, but long-term cardiac effects were studied later in life, with the median age of the study population being 21.5 years.[110,111]

Bradycardia has been reported in an 11 year-old boy, caused by sinus node involvement; he recovered after treatment of his JDM, without any specific drug for bradycardia.[112] Involvement of the papillary muscles has been reported in a patient with JDM with positive anti–CADM-140 antibody.[113] Increased PR interval and congestive heart failure have also been described. Regarding pathologic characteristics, a mild interstitial inflammatory infiltrate and focal fibrosis were revealed in autopsy studies performed in 2 children.[114]

EHLERS-DANLOS SYNDROMES

The Ehlers-Danlos syndromes (EDS) comprise a spectrum of multisystemic manifestations that can affect the skin, ligaments, joints, blood vessels, and internal organs. Ehlers- Danlos syndromes are classified into 3 general categories: classic (EDS I, II), hypermobile (EDS III), and vascular (EDS IV).[115]

The most severe cardiovascular complications have been reported in patients with the vascular type of EDS. In this form, spontaneous rupture of vessels can occur, even without the formation of aneurysm or dissection.[116] Vessels most prone to rupture are the abdominal aorta and its branches, the great vessels of the aortic arch, and the large arteries of the limbs.[117]

Aortic root dilatation is a common finding in EDS, present in 33% of patients with the classic form and 17% with the hypermobile form. Aortic dilatation is more common in young children compared with older children and adults.[118] This finding was supported by newer studies, which also showed that children with EDS and aortic root dilatation can have normalization of their aortic root size. A proposed mechanism for this phenomenon is stiffening of the aortic tissue with age, in the same way that joints stiffen with age.[119,120]

MV prolapse was present in 6% and MV regurgitation in 4.8% of 252 patients with the hypermobile or classic form of EDS; only 1 individual was reported to have tricuspid valve prolapse.[119] Regurgitation of mitral, tricuspid, and aortic valves was seen in 21% of another study group, combined with mild thickening or sclerosis of those valves in 16% of subjects. Mildly increased pulmonary blood pressure and elongated heart were observed in the same population, although no established criteria exist for appropriate heart length.[120]

MARFAN SYNDROME

Marfan syndrome is an autosomal dominant disorder affecting multiple body systems, including the heart and blood vessels, eyes, bones, skin, and lungs. The responsible mutation for the disease is localized in the gene FBN1, which encodes the extracellular matrix protein fibrillin-1.[121] FBN1 gene mutations are also associated with other disorders referred as fibrillinopathies, including the neonatal Marfan syndrome and the isolated ascending aortic aneurysm.[122] In the population bearing the FBN1 mutation, the percentage of patients with aortic dilatation increases with age and reaches 96% by the age of 60 years. Although aortic events before the age of 20 years are rare, their occurrence increases to 75% by the age of 60 years, with risk being higher for men compared with women.[122] The primary cause of death in patients with Marfan syndrome is cardiovascular collapse caused by aortic dissection.

Fibrillin-1 is a component of microfibrils of the extracellular matrix, and it helps maintain structural integrity and confers elasticity to the arterial wall by linking vascular smooth muscle cells to elastin fibrils. Abnormal or absent fibrillin-1 results in impaired coordination of elastic tension. Fibrillin-1 plays an important role in the regulation of TGF-β and matrix metalloproteinases. A deficiency of fibrillin-1 may lead to ineffective tissue repair because of intense elastolysis and increased TGF-β expression, with a consequence of aortic medial degeneration.[123] TGF-β levels are higher in patients with Marfan syndrome, and increased levels of the molecule are correlated with a large aortic root diameter.[124] A small percentage of patients with Marfan syndrome do not possess a mutation in the FBN1 gene, and mutations of the TGF-β receptor-2 gene have also been linked to the Marfan phenotype.[125,126]

Aortic root aneurysm/dissection is the prominent cardiac manifestation of Marfan syndrome and, along with ectopia lentis and FBN1 mutation, count as criteria for the diagnosis according to the revised Ghent criteria. MV prolapse contributes to the systemic score of the Ghent criteria, which is used to document systemic involvement of Marfan syndrome.[127]

The abnormality of the MV includes redundant elongation of one or both valve leaflets, often accompanied by myxomatous thickening. Prolapse and regurgitation are the functional sequelae of these structural abnormalities.[128] It seems that the prevalence of MV prolapse and regurgitation also increases with age. In neonatal Marfan syndrome, MV prolapse and regurgitation are frequently present, with mitral regurgitation being the leading cause of morbidity.[128] An inverse correlation between the age of onset of Marfan syndrome and prevalence of MV prolapse has been revealed.[129] Left myocardial involvement in the presence of aortic insufficiency and/or mitral regurgitation is expected, but the presence of primary myocardial impairment is debatable both in adults and children.[130] Fibrillin-1 is also present in the extracellular matrix of the myocardium and can affect TGF-β expression. Ventricular function can be affected, which has been shown in studies evaluating systolic and diastolic function, irrespective of aortic elasticity or dilatation.[131,132] Abnormalities of repolarization and ventricular arrhythmias have also been reported secondary to increased left ventricular size and MV prolapse.[133]

Although data are limited and conflicting, β-blockers are first-line therapy for the prevention of cardiovascular complications. The rational of their use is the reduction of hemodynamic stress of the aorta. Nevertheless, propranolol has not been shown to be beneficial in decreasing aortic dissection or aortic rupture incidence. Aortic medial degeneration has been found to be prevented by doxycycline, statins, ACE inhibitors, and angiotensin I receptor inhibitors by modulating TGF-β activity.[123] Patients with Marfan syndrome should carefully select the type and level of physical activity, because there is always the risk of a cardiovascular event.[134]

SYSTEMIC JUVENILE IDIOPATHIC ARTHRITIS

Systemic juvenile idiopathic arthritis (JIA), the least common type of chronic arthritis in childhood, is characterized by at least 2 weeks of fever, chronic arthritis in at least one joint, and is accompanied by an evanescent rash, generalized lymphadenopathy, hepatosplenomegaly, or serositis.[135] Cardiac involvement, including pericarditis, myocarditis, and endocarditis, can be seen as a feature of systemic JIA but is extremely rare, as with other subtypes of JIA.

Pericarditis is the most common cardiac complication of systemic JIA. Although the prevalence of overt pericarditis has been estimated at 7% across all subtypes of JIA, up to 45% of autopsies of patients with JIA have revealed evidence of subclinical pericarditis,[136] suggesting that asymptomatic pericarditis is more prevalent. Pericarditis is most common during periods of active disease flare but can occur anytime during the disease course and may even precede the onset of arthritis. When pericarditis is clinically apparent, symptoms (chest pain, dyspnea, worsening when supine) and physical examination findings (tachycardia, muffled heart sounds, friction rub) are typical of those seen with other types of pericarditis.

Although most cases of pericarditis in systemic JIA are insidious and chronic, cardiac tamponade has been described in both systemic JIA and adult-onset Still disease. At least 11 pediatric cases of tamponade have been reported, including tamponade as the presenting feature of systemic JIA.[137] Tamponade is characterized as acute cardiopulmonary decompensation associated with rapid accumulation of fluid in the pericardial sac, jugular venous distention, and pulsus paradoxus. Urgent pericardiocentesis is typically necessary, and further treatment is designed to treat the underlying inflammatory disease.

Myocarditis has been reported in systemic JIA but is much rarer than pericarditis; the two conditions can also coexist. Myocarditis can lead to cardiomegaly and congestive heart failure.[138,139] A small number of cases of endocarditis have been reported in patients with systemic JIA, typically occurring years after the onset of initial systemic arthritis.[140,141]

Therapy for cardiac involvement in systemic JIA should involve treatment of the underlying disease and systemic inflammatory state and typically includes nonsteroidal antiinflammatory drugs, corticosteroids, disease-modifying drugs, and biologic therapies targeting TNF-α, IL-1, and IL-6.

REFERENCES

1. Newburger JW, Takahashi M, Gerber MA, et al. Diagnosis, treatment, and long-term management of Kawasaki disease: a statement for health professionals from the Committee on Rheumatic Fever, Endocarditis, and Kawasaki Disease, Council on Cardiovascular Disease in the Young, American Heart Association. Pediatrics 2004;114(6):1708–33.
2. Uehara R, Belay ED. Epidemiology of Kawasaki disease in Asia, Europe, and the United States. J Epidemiol 2012;22(2):79–85.
3. Yim D, Curtis N, Cheung M, et al. Update on Kawasaki disease: epidemiology, aetiology and pathogenesis. J Paediatr Child Health 2013;49(9):704–8. http://dx.doi.org/10.1111/jpc.12172.
4. Yim D, Curtis N, Cheung M, et al. An update on Kawasaki disease II: clinical features, diagnosis, treatment and outcomes. J Paediatr Child Health 2013;49(8):614–23.
5. Kentsis A, Shulman A, Ahmed S, et al. Urine proteomics for discovery of improved diagnostic markers of Kawasaki disease. EMBO Mol Med 2013; 5(2):210–20.
6. Luca NJ, Yeung RS. Epidemiology and management of Kawasaki disease. Drugs 2012;72(8):1029–38.
7. Ogata S, Tremoulet AH, Sato Y, et al. Coronary artery outcomes among children with Kawasaki disease in the United States and Japan. Int J Cardiol 2013; 168(4):3825–8.
8. Ha KS, Jang G, Lee J, et al. Incomplete clinical manifestation as a risk factor for coronary artery abnormalities in Kawasaki disease: a meta-analysis. Eur J Pediatr 2013;172(3):343–9.
9. Onouchi Y. Genetics of Kawasaki disease: what we know and don't know. Circ J 2012;76(7):1581–6.
10. Rowley AH. Kawasaki disease: novel insights into etiology and genetic susceptibility. Annu Rev Med 2011;62:69–77.

11. Tacke CE, Burgner D, Kuipers IM, et al. Management of acute and refractory Kawasaki disease. Expert Rev Anti Infect Ther 2012;10(10):1203–15.
12. Dominguez SR, Anderson MS. Advances in the treatment of Kawasaki disease. Curr Opin Pediatr 2013;25(1):103–9.
13. Manlhiot C, Niedra E, McCrindle BW. Long-term management of Kawasaki disease: implications for the adult patient. Pediatr Neonatol 2013;54(1):12–21.
14. Seckeler MD, Hoke TR. The worldwide epidemiology of acute rheumatic fever and rheumatic heart disease. Clin Epidemiol 2011;3:67–84.
15. Carapetis JR, Steer AC, Mulholland EK, et al. The global burden of group A streptococcal diseases. Lancet Infect Dis 2005;5(11):685–94.
16. Carapetis JR, McDonald M, Wilson NJ. Acute rheumatic fever. Lancet 2005; 366(9480):155–68.
17. Oen K. Comparative epidemiology of the rheumatic diseases in children. Curr Opin Rheumatol 2000;12(5):410–4.
18. Steer AC, Carapetis JR. Acute rheumatic fever and rheumatic heart disease in indigenous populations. Pediatr Clin North Am 2009;56(6):1401–19.
19. Negi PC, Kanwar A, Chauhan R, et al. Epidemiological trends of RF/RHD in school children of Shimla in north India. Indian J Med Res 2013;137(6): 1121–7.
20. Milne RJ, Lennon DR, Stewart JM, et al. Incidence of acute rheumatic fever in New Zealand children and youth. J Paediatr Child Health 2012;48(8):685–91.
21. Longo-Mbenza B, Bayekula M, Ngiyulu R, et al. Survey of rheumatic heart disease in school children of Kinshasa town. Int J Cardiol 1998;63(3):287–94.
22. Tani LY, Veasy LG, Minich LL, et al. Rheumatic fever in children younger than 5 years: is the presentation different? Pediatrics 2003;112(5):1065–8.
23. Chockalingam A, Prabhakar D, Dorairajan S, et al. Rheumatic heart disease occurrence, patterns and clinical correlates in children aged less than five years. J Heart Valve Dis 2004;13(1):11–4.
24. Breda L, Marzetti V, Gaspari S, et al. Population-based study of incidence and clinical characteristics of rheumatic fever in Abruzzo, central Italy, 2000-2009. J Pediatr 2012;160(5):832–6.e1.
25. Cunningham MW. Pathogenesis of group A streptococcal infections. Clin Microbiol Rev 2000;13(3):470–511.
26. Lymbury RS, Olive C, Powell KA, et al. Induction of autoimmune valvulitis in Lewis rats following immunization with peptides from the conserved region of group A streptococcal M protein. J Autoimmun 2003;20(3):211–7.
27. Oldstone MB. Molecular mimicry and immune-mediated diseases. FASEB J 1998;12(13):1255–65.
28. Barnett LA, Fujinami RS. Molecular mimicry: a mechanism for autoimmune injury. FASEB J 1992;6(3):840–4.
29. Kaplan EL, Johnson DR, Cleary PP. Group A streptococcal serotypes isolated from patients and sibling contacts during the resurgence of rheumatic fever in the United States in the mid-1980s. J Infect Dis 1989;159(1):101–3.
30. Tandon R, Sharma M, Chandrashekhar Y, et al. Revisiting the pathogenesis of rheumatic fever and carditis. Nat Rev Cardiol 2013;10(3):171–7.
31. Cunningham MW. Autoimmunity and molecular mimicry in the pathogenesis of post-streptococcal heart disease. Front Biosci 2003;8:s533–43.
32. Adderson EE, Shikhman AR, Ward KE, et al. Molecular analysis of polyreactive monoclonal antibodies from rheumatic carditis: human anti-N-acetylglucosamine/anti-myosin antibody V region genes. J Immunol 1998; 161(4):2020–31.

33. Luo YH, Chuang WJ, Wu JJ, et al. Molecular mimicry between streptococcal pyrogenic exotoxin B and endothelial cells. Lab Invest 2010;90(10):1492–506.
34. Scalzi V, Hadi HA, Alessandri C, et al. Anti-endothelial cell antibodies in rheumatic heart disease. Clin Exp Immunol 2010;161(3):570–5.
35. Delunardo F, Scalzi V, Capozzi A, et al. Streptococcal-vimentin cross-reactive antibodies induce microvascular cardiac endothelial proinflammatory phenotype in rheumatic heart disease. Clin Exp Immunol 2013;173(3):419–29.
36. Dinkla K, Rohde M, Jansen WT, et al. Rheumatic fever-associated *Streptococcus pyogenes* isolates aggregate collagen. J Clin Invest 2003;111(12): 1905–12.
37. Dinkla K, Talay SR, Morgelin M, et al. Crucial role of the CB3-region of collagen IV in PARF-induced acute rheumatic fever. PLoS One 2009;4(3):e4666.
38. Caughey DE, Douglas R, Wilson W, et al. HL-A antigens in Europeans and Maoris with rheumatic fever and rheumatic heart disease. J Rheumatol 1975; 2(3):319–22.
39. Engel ME, Stander R, Vogel J, et al. Genetic susceptibility to acute rheumatic fever: a systematic review and meta-analysis of twin studies. PLoS One 2011; 6(9):e25326.
40. Azevedo PM, Pereira RR, Guilherme L. Understanding rheumatic fever. Rheumatol Int 2012;32(5):1113–20.
41. Gupta U, Mishra A, Rathore SS, et al. Association of angiotensin I-converting enzyme gene insertion/deletion polymorphism with rheumatic heart disease in Indian population and meta-analysis. Mol Cell Biochem 2013;382(1–2): 75–82.
42. Col-Araz N, Pehlivan S, Baspinar O, et al. Role of cytokine gene (IFN-gamma, TNF-alpha, TGF-beta 1, IL-6, and IL-10) polymorphisms in pathogenesis of acute rheumatic fever in Turkish children. Eur J Pediatr 2012;171(7): 1103–8.
43. Jones TD. The diagnosis of rheumatic fever. JAMA 1944;126(8):481–4.
44. Jones criteria (modified) for guidance in the diagnosis of rheumatic fever. Public Health Rep 1956;71(7):672–4.
45. Jones criteria (revised) for guidance in the diagnosis of rheumatic fever. Circulation 1965;32(4):664–8.
46. Jones criteria (revised) for guidance in the diagnosis of rheumatic fever. Circulation 1984;69(1):204A–8A.
47. Guidelines for the diagnosis of rheumatic fever. Jones criteria, 1992 update. Special Writing Group of the Committee on Rheumatic Fever, Endocarditis, and Kawasaki Disease of the Council on Cardiovascular Disease in the Young of the American Heart Association. JAMA 1992;268(15):2069–73.
48. Chagani HS, Aziz K. Clinical profile of acute rheumatic fever in Pakistan. Cardiol Young 2003;13(1):28–35.
49. Pereira BA, da Silva NA, Andrade LE, et al. Jones criteria and underdiagnosis of rheumatic fever. Indian J Pediatr 2007;74(2):117–21.
50. Grover A, Dhawan A, Iyengar SD, et al. Epidemiology of rheumatic fever and rheumatic heart disease in a rural community in northern India. Bull World Health Organ 1993;71(1):59–66.
51. Steer AC, Kado J, Jenney AW, et al. Acute rheumatic fever and rheumatic heart disease in Fiji: prospective surveillance, 2005-2007. Med J Aust 2009;190(3): 133–5.
52. Caldas AM, Terreri MT, Moises VA, et al. What is the true frequency of carditis in acute rheumatic fever? A prospective clinical and Doppler blind study of 56

children with up to 60 months of follow-up evaluation. Pediatr Cardiol 2008; 29(6):1048–53.

53. Rayamajhi A, Sharma D, Shakya U. Clinical, laboratory and echocardiographic profile of acute rheumatic fever in Nepali children. Ann Trop Paediatr 2007; 27(3):169–77.

54. Olgunturk R, Canter B, Tunaoglu FS, et al. Review of 609 patients with rheumatic fever in terms of revised and updated Jones criteria. Int J Cardiol 2006;112(1): 91–8.

55. Wilson N. Rheumatic heart disease in indigenous populations–New Zealand experience. Heart Lung Circ 2010;19(5–6):282–8.

56. Figueroa FE, Fernandez MS, Valdes P, et al. Prospective comparison of clinical and echocardiographic diagnosis of rheumatic carditis: long term follow up of patients with subclinical disease. Heart 2001;85(4):407–10.

57. Abernethy M, Bass N, Sharpe N, et al. Doppler echocardiography and the early diagnosis of carditis in acute rheumatic fever. Aust N Z J Med 1994;24(5):530–5.

58. Majeed HA, Yousof AM, Khuffash FA, et al. The natural-history of acute rheumatic-fever in Kuwait – A prospective 6 year follow-up report. J Chronic Dis 1986;39(5):361–9.

59. Olgunturk R, Aydin GB, Tunaoglu FS, et al. Rheumatic heart disease prevalence among schoolchildren in Ankara, Turkey. Turk J Pediatr 1999;41(2):201–6.

60. Orun UA, Ceylan O, Bilici M, et al. Acute rheumatic fever in the central Anatolia region of Turkey: a 30-year experience in a single center. Eur J Pediatr 2012; 171(2):361–8.

61. Hashkes PJ, Tauber T, Somekh E, et al. Naproxen as an alternative to aspirin for the treatment of arthritis of rheumatic fever: a randomized trial. J Pediatr 2003; 143(3):399–401.

62. Barash J. Rheumatic fever and post-group a streptococcal arthritis in children. Curr Infect Dis Rep 2013;15(3):263–8.

63. Herdy GV, Gomes RS, Silva AE, et al. Follow-up of rheumatic carditis treated with steroids. Cardiol Young 2012;22(3):263–9.

64. Cilliers A, Manyemba J, Adler AJ, et al. Anti-inflammatory treatment for carditis in acute rheumatic fever. Cochrane Database Syst Rev 2012;(6):CD003176.

65. Voss LM, Wilson NJ, Neutze JM, et al. Intravenous immunoglobulin in acute rheumatic fever – A randomized controlled trial. Circulation 2001;103(3):401–6.

66. Gerber MA, Baltimore RS, Eaton CB, et al. Prevention of rheumatic fever and diagnosis and treatment of acute streptococcal pharyngitis: a scientific statement from the American Heart Association Rheumatic Fever, Endocarditis, and Kawasaki Disease Committee of the Council on Cardiovascular Disease in the Young, the Interdisciplinary Council on Functional Genomics and Translational Biology, and the Interdisciplinary Council on Quality of Care and Outcomes Research: endorsed by the American Academy of Pediatrics. Circulation 2009;119(11):1541–51.

67. Crea MA, Mortimer EA Jr. The nature of scarlatinal arthritis. Pediatrics 1959; 23(5):879–84.

68. van der Helm-van Mil AH. Acute rheumatic fever and poststreptococcal reactive arthritis reconsidered. Curr Opin Rheumatol 2010;22(4):437–42.

69. Riise OR, Handeland KS, Cvancarova M, et al. Incidence and characteristics of arthritis in Norwegian children: a population-based study. Pediatrics 2008; 121(2):e299–306.

70. Mackie SL, Keat A. Poststreptococcal reactive arthritis: what is it and how do we know? Rheumatology 2004;43(8):949–54.

71. Tutar E, Atalay S, Yilmaz E, et al. Poststreptococcal reactive arthritis in children: is it really a different entity from rheumatic fever? Rheumatol Int 2002;22(2):80–3.

72. Sarakbi HA, Hammoudeh M, Kanjar I, et al. Poststreptococcal reactive arthritis and the association with tendonitis, tenosynovitis, and enthesitis. J Clin Rheumatol 2010;16(1):3–6.

73. van Bemmel JM, Delgado V, Holman ER, et al. No increased risk of valvular heart disease in adult poststreptococcal reactive arthritis. Arthritis Rheum 2009;60(4):987–93.

74. Moorthy LN, Gaur S, Peterson MG, et al. Poststreptococcal reactive arthritis in children: a retrospective study. Clin Pediatr 2009;48(2):174–82.

75. Decunto CL, Giannini EH, Fink CW, et al. Prognosis of children with poststreptococcal reactive arthritis. Pediatr Infect Dis J 1988;7(10):683–6.

76. Ayoub EM, Ahmed S. Update on complications of group A streptococcal infections. Curr Probl Pediatr 1997;27(3):90–101.

77. Chang C. Neonatal autoimmune diseases: a critical review. J Autoimmun 2012; 38(23):J223–38.

78. Inzinger M, Salmhofer W, Binder B. Neonatal lupus erythematosus and its clinical variability. J Dtsch Dermatol Ges 2012;10(6):407–11.

79. Izmirly PM, Buyon JP, Saxena A. Neonatal lupus: advances in understanding pathogenesis and identifying treatments of cardiac disease. Curr Opin Rheumatol 2012;24(5):466–72.

80. Karnabi E, Qu Y, Mancarella S, et al. Rescue and worsening of congenital heart block-associated electrocardiographic abnormalities in two transgenic mice. J Cardiovasc Electrophysiol 2011;22(8):922–30.

81. Briassouli P, Komissarova EV, Clancy RM, et al. Role of the urokinase plasminogen activator receptor in mediating impaired efferocytosis of anti-SSA/Ro-bound apoptotic cardiocytes: implications in the pathogenesis of congenital heart block. Circ Res 2010;107(3):374–87.

82. Reed JH, Clancy RM, Purcell AW, et al. Beta-2-glycoprotein I and protection from anti-SSA/Ro60-associated cardiac manifestations of neonatal lupus. J Immunol 2011;187(1):520–6.

83. Briassouli P, Rifkin D, Clancy RM, et al. Binding of anti-SSA antibodies to apoptotic fetal cardiocytes stimulates urokinase plasminogen activator (uPA)/uPA receptor-dependent activation of TGF-beta and potentiates fibrosis. J Immunol 2011;187(10):5392–401.

84. Izmirly PM, Saxena A, Kim MY, et al. Maternal and fetal factors associated with mortality and morbidity in a multi-racial/ethnic registry of anti-SSA/Ro-associated cardiac neonatal lupus. Circulation 2011;124(18):1927–35.

85. Brucato A, Frassi M, Franceschini F, et al. Risk of congenital complete heart block in newborns of mothers with anti-Ro/SSA antibodies detected by counterimmunoelectrophoresis: a prospective study of 100 women. Arthritis Rheum 2001;44(8):1832–5.

86. Llanos C, Izmirly PM, Katholi M, et al. Recurrence rates of cardiac manifestations associated with neonatal lupus and maternal/fetal risk factors. Arthritis Rheum 2009;60(10):3091–7.

87. Zhao H, Cuneo BF, Strasburger JF, et al. Electrophysiological characteristics of fetal atrioventricular block. J Am Coll Cardiol 2008;51(1):77–84.

88. Hornberger LK, Al Rajaa N. Spectrum of cardiac involvement in neonatal lupus. Scand J Immunol 2010;72:189–97.

89. Cimaz R, Meroni PL, Brucato A, et al. Concomitant disappearance of electrocardiographic abnormalities and of acquired maternal autoantibodies during the

first year of life in infants who had QT interval prolongation and anti-SSA/Ro positivity without congenital heart block at birth. Arthritis Rheum 2003;48(1):266–8.
90. Costedoat-Chalumeau N, Amoura Z, Lupoglazoff JM, et al. Outcome of pregnancies in patients with anti-SSA/Ro antibodies: a study of 165 pregnancies, with special focus on electrocardiographic variations in the children and comparison with a control group. Arthritis Rheum 2004;50(10):3187–94.
91. Nield LE, Silverman ED, Taylor GP, et al. Maternal anti-Ro and anti-La antibody-associated endocardial fibroelastosis. Circulation 2002;105(7):843–8.
92. Nield LE, Silverman ED, Smallhorn JF, et al. Endocardial fibroelastosis associated with maternal anti-Ro and anti-La antibodies in the absence of atrioventricular block. J Am Coll Cardiol 2002;40(4):796–802.
93. Guettrot-Imbert G, Cohen L, Fermont L, et al. A new presentation of neonatal lupus: 5 cases of isolated mild endocardial fibroelastosis associated with maternal anti-SSA/Ro and Anti-SSB/La antibodies. J Rheumatol 2011;38(2):378–86.
94. Jaeggi ET, Hamilton RM, Silverman ED, et al. Outcome of children with fetal, neonatal or childhood diagnosis of isolated congenital atrioventricular block. A single institution's experience of 30 years. J Am Coll Cardiol 2002;39(1):130–7.
95. Moak JP, Barron KS, Hougen TJ, et al. Congenital heart block: development of late-onset cardiomyopathy, a previously underappreciated sequelae. J Am Coll Cardiol 2001;37(1):238–42.
96. Saleeb S, Copel J, Friedman D, et al. Comparison of treatment with fluorinated glucocorticoids to the natural history of autoantibody-associated congenital heart block: retrospective review of the research registry for neonatal lupus. Arthritis Rheum 1999;42(11):2335–45.
97. Eronen M, Siren MK, Ekblad H, et al. Short- and long-term outcome of children with congenital complete heart block diagnosed in utero or as a newborn. Pediatrics 2000;106(1 Pt 1):86–91.
98. Llanos C, Friedman DM, Saxena A, et al. Anatomical and pathological findings in hearts from fetuses and infants with cardiac manifestations of neonatal lupus. Rheumatology (Oxford) 2012;51(6):1086–92.
99. Buyon JP, Clancy RM, Friedman DM. Cardiac manifestations of neonatal lupus erythematosus: guidelines to management, integrating clues from the bench and bedside. Nat Clin Pract Rheumatol 2009;5(3):139–48.
100. Friedman DM, Kim MY, Copel JA, et al. Prospective evaluation of fetuses with autoimmune-associated congenital heart block followed in the PR Interval and Dexamethasone Evaluation (PRIDE) study. Am J Cardiol 2009;103(8):1102–6.
101. Friedman DM, Llanos C, Izmirly PM, et al. Evaluation of fetuses in a study of intravenous immunoglobulin as preventive therapy for congenital heart block: results of a multicenter, prospective, open-label clinical trial. Arthritis Rheum 2010;62(4):1138–46.
102. Pisoni CN, Brucato A, Ruffatti A, et al. Failure of intravenous immunoglobulin to prevent congenital heart block: findings of a multicenter, prospective, observational study. Arthritis Rheum 2010;62(4):1147–52.
103. Izmirly PM, Kim MY, Llanos C, et al. Evaluation of the risk of anti-SSA/Ro-SSB/La antibody-associated cardiac manifestations of neonatal lupus in fetuses of mothers with systemic lupus erythematosus exposed to hydroxychloroquine. Ann Rheum Dis 2010;69(10):1827–30.
104. Izmirly PM, Costedoat-Chalumeau N, Pisoni CN, et al. Maternal use of hydroxychloroquine is associated with a reduced risk of recurrent anti-SSA/Ro-antibody-

associated cardiac manifestations of neonatal lupus. Circulation 2012;126(1):
76–82.

105. Trucco SM, Jaeggi E, Cuneo B, et al. Use of intravenous gamma globulin and
corticosteroids in the treatment of maternal autoantibody-mediated cardiomyopathy. J Am Coll Cardiol 2011;57(6):715–23.

106. Feldman BM, Rider LG, Reed AM, et al. Juvenile dermatomyositis and other
idiopathic inflammatory myopathies of childhood. Lancet 2008;371(9631):
2201–12.

107. Zhang L, Wang GC, Ma L, et al. Cardiac involvement in adult polymyositis or
dermatomyositis: a systematic review. Clin Cardiol 2012;35(11):686–91.

108. Shehata R, al-Mayouf S, al-Dalaan A, et al. Juvenile dermatomyositis: clinical
profile and disease course in 25 patients. Clin Exp Rheumatol 1999;17(1):
115–8.

109. Constantin T, Ponyi A, Orban I, et al. National registry of patients with juvenile
idiopathic inflammatory myopathies in Hungary–clinical characteristics and disease course of 44 patients with juvenile dermatomyositis. Autoimmunity 2006;
39(3):223–32.

110. Schwartz T, Sanner H, Husebye T, et al. Cardiac dysfunction in juvenile dermatomyositis: a case-control study. Ann Rheum Dis 2011;70(5):766–71.

111. Schwartz T, Sanner H, Gjesdal O, et al. In juvenile dermatomyositis, cardiac systolic dysfunction is present after long-term follow-up and is predicted by sustained early skin activity. Ann Rheum Dis 2013. [Epub ahead of print].

112. Karaca NE, Aksu G, Yeniay BS, et al. Juvenile dermatomyositis with a rare
and remarkable complication: sinus bradycardia. Rheumatol Int 2006;27(2):
179–82.

113. Sakurai N, Nagai K, Tsutsumi H, et al. Anti-CADM-140 antibody-positive juvenile
dermatomyositis with rapidly progressive interstitial lung disease and cardiac
involvement. J Rheumatol 2011;38(5):963–4.

114. Haupt HM, Hutchins GM. The heart and cardiac conduction system in
polymyositis-dermatomyositis: a clinicopathologic study of 16 autopsied patients. Am J Cardiol 1982;50(5):998–1006.

115. Beighton P, De Paepe A, Steinmann B, et al. Ehlers-Danlos syndromes: revised
nosology, Villefranche, 1997. Ehlers-Danlos National Foundation (USA) and
Ehlers-Danlos Support Group (UK). Am J Med Genet 1998;77(1):31–7.

116. Beridze N, Frishman WH. Vascular Ehlers-Danlos syndrome: pathophysiology,
diagnosis, and prevention and treatment of its complications. Cardiol Rev
2012;20(1):4–7.

117. De Paepe A, Malfait F. Bleeding and bruising in patients with Ehlers-Danlos syndrome and other collagen vascular disorders. Br J Haematol 2004;127(5):
491–500.

118. Wenstrup RJ, Meyer RA, Lyle JS, et al. Prevalence of aortic root dilation in the
Ehlers-Danlos syndrome. Genet Med 2002;4(3):112–7.

119. Atzinger CL, Meyer RA, Khoury PR, et al. Cross-sectional and longitudinal
assessment of aortic root dilation and valvular anomalies in hypermobile and
classic Ehlers-Danlos syndrome. J Pediatr 2011;158(5):826–30.e1.

120. McDonnell NB, Gorman BL, Mandel KW, et al. Echocardiographic findings in
classical and hypermobile Ehlers-Danlos syndromes. Am J Med Genet A
2006;140(2):129–36.

121. Pearson GD, Devereux R, Loeys B, et al. Report of the National Heart, Lung, and
Blood Institute and National Marfan Foundation Working Group on research in
Marfan syndrome and related disorders. Circulation 2008;118(7):785–91.

122. Detaint D, Faivre L, Collod-Beroud G, et al. Cardiovascular manifestations in men and women carrying a FBN1 mutation. Eur Heart J 2010;31(18):2223–9.
123. Hartog AW, Franken R, Zwinderman AH, et al. Current and future pharmacological treatment strategies with regard to aortic disease in Marfan syndrome. Expert Opin Pharmacother 2012;13(5):647–62.
124. Franken R, den Hartog AW, de Waard V, et al. Circulating transforming growth factor-beta as a prognostic biomarker in Marfan syndrome. Int J Cardiol 2013; 168(3):2441–6.
125. Akhurst RJ. TGF beta signaling in health and disease. Nat Genet 2004;36(8): 790–2.
126. Mizuguchi T, Collod-Beroud G, Akiyama T, et al. Heterozygous TGFBR2 mutations in Marfan syndrome. Nat Genet 2004;36(8):855–60.
127. Loeys BL, Dietz HC, Braverman AC, et al. The revised Ghent nosology for the Marfan syndrome. J Med Genet 2010;47(7):476–85.
128. Judge DP, Rouf R, Habashi J, et al. Mitral valve disease in Marfan syndrome and related disorders. J Cardiovasc Transl Res 2011;4(6):741–7.
129. Faivre L, Masurel-Paulet A, Collod-Beroud G, et al. Clinical and molecular study of 320 children with Marfan syndrome and related type I fibrillinopathies in a series of 1009 probands with pathogenic FBN1 mutations. Pediatrics 2009;123(1): 391–8.
130. Kiotsekoglou A, Sutherland GR, Moggridge JC, et al. The unravelling of primary myocardial impairment in Marfan syndrome by modern echocardiography. Heart 2009;95(19):1561–6.
131. de Witte P, Aalberts JJ, Radonic T, et al. Intrinsic biventricular dysfunction in Marfan syndrome. Heart 2011;97(24):2063–8.
132. Das BB, Taylor AL, Yetman AT. Left ventricular diastolic dysfunction in children and young adults with Marfan syndrome. Pediatr Cardiol 2006;27(2):256–8.
133. Yetman AT, Bornemeier RA, McCrindle BW. Long-term outcome in patients with Marfan syndrome: is aortic dissection the only cause of sudden death? J Am Coll Cardiol 2003;41(2):329–32.
134. Maron BJ, Chaitman BR, Ackerman MJ, et al. Recommendations for physical activity and recreational sports participation for young patients with genetic cardiovascular diseases. Circulation 2004;109(22):2807–16.
135. Petty RE, Southwood TR, Manners P, et al. ILAR classification of juvenile idiopathic arthritis, second revision, Edmonton, 2001. J Rheumatol 2004;31:390–2.
136. Lietman P, Bywaters EG. Pericarditis in juvenile rheumatoid arthritis. Pediatrics 1963;32:855–60.
137. Baszis KW, Singh G, White AJ, et al. Recurrent cardiac tamponade in a child with newly diagnosed systemic-onset juvenile idiopathic arthritis. J Clin Rheumatol 2012;18:304–6.
138. Goldenberg J, Ferraz MB, Pessoa AP, et al. Symptomatic cardiac involvement in juvenile rheumatoid arthritis. Int J Cardiol 1992;34:57–62.
139. Miller JJ 3rd, French JW. Myocarditis in juvenile rheumatoid arthritis. Am J Dis Child 1977;131:205–9.
140. Kramer PH, Imboden JB Jr, Waldman FM, et al. Severe aortic insufficiency in juvenile chronic arthritis. Am J Med 1983;74:1088–91.
141. Heyd J, Glaser J. Early occurrence of aortic valve regurgitation in a youth with systemic-onset juvenile rheumatoid arthritis. Am J Med 1990;89:123–4.

Systemic Sclerosis and the Heart

John L. Parks, MD[a], Marian H. Taylor, MD[a], Laura P. Parks, MD[b],
Richard M. Silver, MD[b],*

KEYWORDS

- Scleroderma • Systemic sclerosis • Heart disease • Pericarditis
- Myocardial fibrosis • Conduction abnormalities

KEY POINTS

- Although definitive therapy for heart disease related to systemic sclerosis (SSc) has been elusive, novel approaches are being explored.
- It is hoped that hematopoietic stem cell transplantation might demonstrate improvement in heart disease related to SSc, but this has not been investigated to date.
- Cyclophosphamide and imatinib are other potential therapies for patients with SSc, but data regarding efficacy in heart disease associated with SSc are also lacking.
- The cardiac disease associated with scleroderma can present in many forms and is often clinically silent until significant organ dysfunction has ensued.
- As clinical awareness and diagnostic methods have improved, earlier detection and treatment are both feasible and advisable.

INTRODUCTION

In 1945, Goetz and Berne[1] characterized scleroderma as a disease with progressive cutaneous and multi-organ involvement, coining the term *systemic sclerosis* (SSc). Widespread sclerosis of the skin, with other concurrent ailments, had been noted earlier by many scholars and was initially defined by Curzio[2] in the eighteenth century. It was the works by Heine[3] in 1926 and Weiss and Warren[4] in 1943 that laid a foundation for the disease's involvement of the heart. These investigators described scleroderma in association with cardiac findings and postulated a direct relationship rather than a mere association. SSc has now been recognized as a disease that often has cardiac involvement manifested by multiple processes with potentially serious implications for patients. The myriad of presentations includes involvement of the pericardium, myocardium, conduction system, and vasculature. Weiss, Stead, and Warren's[3] series in 1943 was a landmark investigation, describing 9 patients with cutaneous

Disclosures: none.
[a] Division of Cardiology, Medical University of South Carolina, 96 Jonathan Lucas Street, Charleston, SC 29425, USA; [b] Division of Rheumatology & Immunology, Medical University of South Carolina, 96 Jonathan Lucas Street, Charleston, SC 29425, USA
* Corresponding author. 96 Jonathan Lucas Street, Suite 816 CSB, Charleston, SC 29425.
E-mail address: silverr@musc.edu

Rheum Dis Clin N Am 40 (2014) 87–102
http://dx.doi.org/10.1016/j.rdc.2013.10.007
0889-857X/14/$ – see front matter © 2014 Elsevier Inc. All rights reserved.

findings of scleroderma associated with concurrent cardiac disease. The patients described symptoms of heart failure, and the investigators suspected a direct relationship related to widespread fibrosis of both the skin and heart.[5] Myocardial fibrosis caused directly by SSc, not related to pulmonary or renal complications, was initially debated. A seminal study by Bulkley and colleagues[6] of 52 autopsy cases at The Johns Hopkins Hospital made significant strides to define primary cardiac involvement in SSc. These investigators identified patients with myocardial fibrosis who were noted to have had significant symptoms of heart failure, angina pectoris, and dysrhythmias. At autopsy they were found to have contraction band necrosis and replacement fibrosis without associated coronary disease and without pulmonary, renal, or systemic vascular disease that would offer a secondary explanation. It was postulated that the myocardial fibrosis was related to a Raynaudlike phenomenon of the microvasculature, leading to ischemia-reperfusion injury with multiple small areas of necrosis and eventual fibrosis. Through extensive study, patchy myocardial fibrosis has been recognized as a hallmark of scleroderma heart disease.

Symptoms of heart failure and underlying myocardial fibrosis are by no means the sole finding of cardiac disease in SSc (**Table 1**). As more investigation has been undertaken, pericardial disease and conduction abnormalities have become more apparent. Both acute pericarditis and chronic pericardial effusion have been described, rarely with effusions causing cardiac tamponade. In a series described by McWhorter and LeRoy[7] in 1974, pericardial involvement was more common than significant myocardial fibrosis at autopsy (62% vs 30%). However, pericardial involvement may often be limited to asymptomatic effusions; clinically significant disease is less common. A wide spectrum of dysrhythmias and conduction abnormalities may be seen in scleroderma, varying from premature ventricular contractions to heart block or potentially fatal ventricular dysrhythmias. James[8] published an autopsy analysis in 1974 of 8 patients with scleroderma and cardiac symptoms that revealed abnormalities in the sinus node, atrioventricular node, His bundle, and small coronary arteries. Widespread narrowing of these small coronary arteries (less than 1 mm diameter) caused by mural fibrosis, endothelial proliferation, and platelet-fibrin clots were thought to be the basis for myocardial fibrosis and also structural abnormalities in the conduction tissue they supplied.[8] These microvascular abnormalities have established a plausible nidus for varying degrees of heart block and dysrhythmias.

The various cardiovascular diseases in scleroderma represent a wide spectrum of clinical entities, varying from asymptomatic processes to those associated with much morbidity and mortality. Although disease-modifying therapy is lacking at this time, early consideration of organ involvement (eg, scleroderma heart disease) may allow treatment of secondary processes and more aggressive management of symptoms. This recognition of cardiac involvement requires attention and interventions led by internists, cardiologists, and rheumatologists.

Table 1 Cardiac manifestations of SSc	
Pericardial	Acute pericarditis, chronic pericarditis, pericardial fibrosis, pericardial effusion, tamponade
Myocardial	Myocardial fibrosis, ventricular diastolic dysfunction, ventricular systolic dysfunction, myocarditis
Conduction system disease	Autonomic dysfunction, heart block, supraventricular dysrhythmia, ventricular dysrhythmia
Vascular	Mural fibrosis, intimal proliferation, platelet-fibrin clotting

INCIDENCE AND PROGNOSIS

Cardiovascular involvement in scleroderma is often unrecognized, making it difficult to estimate the true frequency. Depending on the diagnostic technique used, contemporary reviews suggest a clinical incidence of cardiac involvement in 15% to 35% of patients with SSc.[9] Postmortem study was the initial methodology allowing for the first identification of cardiac disease in scleroderma. Analysis at autopsy likely biases toward those with the most severe systemic processes but allows definitive identification of even occult pathophysiology. Noninvasive studies, such as electrocardiography (ECG), echocardiography, thallium scintigraphy, single-photon emission computed tomography (SPECT), or magnetic resonance imaging (MRI), can identify less clinically apparent processes. Echocardiography and other imaging modalities may also recognize sequelae of other organ system involvement, such as elevated right ventricular pressures secondary to pulmonary hypertension. These modalities may identify patients without symptoms earlier in the disease course, optimizing the opportunity for intervention.

Significant cardiac involvement in SSc portends a poor prognosis. A study by Medsger and Masi[10] in 1973 reported that patients with SSc with clinically apparent cardiac disease had an estimated 5-year mortality as high as 70%. Further analyses propose a lower mortality rate. Although not all of the deaths were related to primary cardiac causes, the findings indicate that cardiac involvement is a harbinger of more aggressive systemic disease. Larger analyses have shown that cardiac-related causes of death account for 14% to 36% of all-cause mortality.[11,12] A recent meta-analysis of 2691 patients with SSc reported an overall mortality rate of 27% at a mean follow-up period of 7.3 years; 29% of deaths were defined as related to cardiac causes.[13]

The skin-thickness-progression rate has also been identified as a method of predicting significant organ involvement, including cardiac disease. Domsic and colleagues[14] demonstrated that severe cardiac involvement was statistically more common in patients with rapid skin thickness progression. Rapid cutaneous progression was associated with severe cardiac disease in 3% of patients versus 1% of patients with a slow skin-thickness-progression rate ($P = .03$). These findings may suggest that patients with rapid skin thickness progression should be monitored more closely for signs or symptoms of cardiac disease.

Although pathologic cardiac involvement has traditionally been associated with diffuse cutaneous SSc (dcSSc), there has been increasing recognition that patients with limited cutaneous SSc (lcSSc) may also have significant cardiac abnormalities. As noninvasive imaging techniques have become more advanced, the identification of cardiac abnormalities in lcSSc has shown to be equal to the incidence in dcSSc. Registry analyses using MRI or echocardiography have demonstrated that the presence of cardiac abnormality is statistically equal in patients with dcSSc and lcSSc.[15,16] However, there is a higher prevalence of symptomatic disease associated with dcSSc.[17]

MYOCARDIAL DISEASE

Myocardial disease is a prominent feature in patients with scleroderma with cardiovascular involvement, with a wide range of manifestations and varying underlying pathophysiology. Microvascular alterations, collagen overproduction, and complex immune system dysregulation lead to ischemic, fibrotic, and inflammatory lesions involving the myocardium (**Fig. 1**).[12,18] These processes may ultimately manifest as ventricular fibrosis (principally recognized as diastolic dysfunction), ventricular systolic dysfunction, myositis, or myocarditis. Although other imaging modalities have been

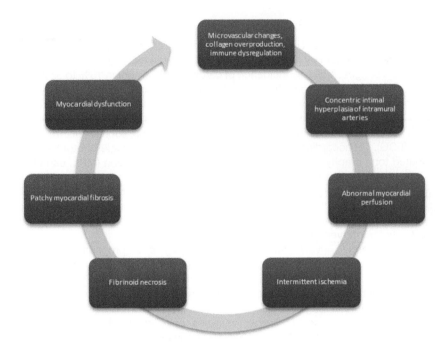

Fig. 1. Proposed mechanism for myocardial fibrosis in SSc.

developed, echocardiography remains the standard method for the assessment of the myocardium largely because of its relative accuracy, reproducibility, sensitivity, and widespread availability. However, innovations in imaging have added new modalities to aid clinicians and may be useful in conjunction with standard techniques (**Box 1**).

Myocardial Fibrosis and Ventricular Diastolic Dysfunction

The pathologic hallmark of SSc cardiac involvement is patchy myocardial fibrosis with a characteristically haphazard distribution of lesions in the myocardium.[19,20] The

---

Box 1
Diagnostic modalities in SSc-related heart disease

ECG

Chest radiography

Doppler echocardiography

Tissue Doppler echocardiography

Echo-derived myocardial strain rate

Thallium perfusion scanning with SPECT

Six-minute walk test

Cardiopulmonary exercise testing

Calcium scoring by computed tomography

MRI

Cardiac catheterization

fibrosis of the myocardium of SSc differs from that observed in atherosclerotic coronary artery disease in that it does not correspond to the regional distribution of a single coronary artery. Ventricular diastolic function is thought to be one of the principal noninvasive measures of myocardial fibrosis. Impaired ventricular filling, synonymous with diastolic dysfunction, has traditionally been identified by means of Doppler echocardiography. Impaired filling may involve either or both ventricles, and multiple studies have demonstrated diastolic dysfunction in patients with SSc.[19,21–24] Impaired ventricular filling represents a stiff or fibrotic ventricle, which may eventually lead to upstream effects, such as atrial enlargement and associated dysrhythmias, pulmonary venous congestion and pulmonary edema, or ventricular systolic dysfunction.

Impaired ventricular filling is more pronounced in patients with SSc with predisposing conditions, such as systemic hypertension, but is often one of the first markers of primary scleroderma heart disease.[19,23,24] Diastolic dysfunction is not limited to the left ventricle; a surprisingly high prevalence of right-sided diastolic abnormalities has been reported in patients regardless of SSc subset. Right ventricular diastolic dysfunction correlates independently with both pulmonary hypertension and left ventricular diastolic dysfunction.[19,24,25] Giunta and colleagues[25] assessed diastolic function by echocardiography in 77 patients with SSc compared with 33 controls; an abnormal right ventricular filling pattern was found in 40% of patients with SSc but not in controls ($P<.001$). These abnormal filling patterns reflect elevated pulmonary pressures, either secondary to left ventricular diastolic dysfunction or pulmonary arterial hypertension. It was concluded that patchy fibrosis impairs the diastolic function of both ventricles, but right ventricular diastolic dysfunction may also represent elevated pulmonary afterload. These studies confirm the frequent occurrence of diastolic dysfunction in patients with SSc regardless of concomitant systemic hypertension or atherosclerotic coronary artery disease.

Ventricular diastolic dysfunction is readily identified using tissue Doppler echocardiography (TDE), which is a relatively new ultrasound technique. TDE allows direct determination of myocardial tissue velocities, patterns of tissue movement, and myocardial strain rate (SR).[26–29] Data obtained from the mitral or tricuspid valve inflow pattern, valve annulus Doppler velocities, and pulmonary venous flow Doppler patterns allows for the identification and staging of diastolic dysfunction. TDE has emerged as a robust indicator of both left and right ventricular contractility and stiffness. Early ventricular diastolic filling velocities gauge ventricular stiffness, which likely correlates with myocardial fibrosis. Ventricular filling velocities have emerged as another useful echo technique for recognizing dysfunction.[30] In the specific context of SSc, combining conventional echocardiography with mitral and tricuspid annular velocity measurements results in greater detection of cardiac complications.[31] Considering the availability of pulsed TDE, it should be considered for routine evaluation of patients with SSc. Because of its usefulness, tissue Doppler study is now commonly a standard component of echocardiography in many centers.

SPECT imaging of thallium perfusion was identified as a modality to demonstrate stress-induced perfusion defects thought to represent fibrotic or microvasculature changes associated with SSc cardiac involvement.[32] The prevalence of cardiac abnormalities identified using exercise or cold provocation SPECT has widely varied, as high as 82% of patients.[33] In comparison, Nakajima and colleagues[34] compared 34 patients with SSc to 16 controls using exercise nongated and rest-gated SPECT and identified minimal perfusion abnormalities in 9 patients, whereas diastolic dysfunction was confirmed in more than half the patients with SSc using echocardiography. Although SPECT seems sensitive to identify potential cardiac abnormalities, the clinical significance of these abnormalities remains uncertain.

Cardiac MRI has emerged as a sensitive technique for identifying cardiac disease in SSc. Imaging techniques include gadolinium-delayed contrast enhancement to evaluate for myocardial fibrosis, T2-weighted imaging to identify inflammatory lesions, and accurate measurements of chamber dimensions and volumes to asses ejection fraction or chamber sizing.[35,36] Cardiac MRI has identified a high incidence of disease that correlates with previous autopsy studies, which may imply a sensitivity advantage over echocardiography. An MRI study of 52 patients from a French center reported some form of cardiac disease in 75%, with equal incidence in dcSSc compared with lcSSc.[15] Although not confirmed with histologic specimens, MRI demonstrated linear midmyocardial delayed contrast enhancement thought to correlate with myocardial fibrosis. Increased uptake with T2-weighted images may suggest myocardial edema and acute inflammation. Ventricular diastolic function and kinetic patterns may be examined with MRI, and right ventricular dysfunction may be more readily identified with MRI compared with echocardiography.[35]

Although conventional echocardiography has been the standard diagnostic modality, echo-derived myocardial SR has been recognized recently as a sensitive method for identifying diastolic dysfunction. SR is a powerful correlate of myocardial contraction and is independent of myocardial translational motion.[26-29] SR may provide a method for identifying myocardial fibrosis at an earlier stage. In one study examining SR, patients with SSc with a normal cardiac examination, pulmonary artery pressure, and radionuclide left ventricular ejection fraction (LVEF) were compared with matched controls[37]; patients with SSc had lower systolic SR and lower diastolic SR than controls. SR may detect reduced left ventricular contractility in the setting of a normal LVEF, allowing for early identification of depressed myocardial contractility.[31,38,39]

There are limited data on therapy for diastolic dysfunction or myocardial fibrosis in SSc. Conventional wisdom suggests that afterload reduction may be beneficial because this is the primary therapeutic strategy in other forms of diastolic dysfunction. However, studies have provided mixed results. One small investigation of ventricular function before and after enalapril therapy found no statistical difference in either patients with SSc or control subjects after 3 months of therapy.[40] In contrast, another study examining the effects of captopril therapy (after at least 11 months) revealed a statistical difference in ventricular function with captopril use.[41] LVEF and markers of diastolic function were statistically improved.

Another target of vasodilator therapy has been the so-called Raynaud phenomena of the microvasculature. In a study using nifedipine (60 mg/d for 14 days), posterior wall systolic SR and diastolic SR increased significantly.[42] Because peak systolic and early diastolic SR are respective indicators of regional contractility and diastolic function, nifedipine is thought to improve myocardial contraction. This conclusion is thought to have significant merit because SR determined by Doppler echocardiography is less load-dependent than other methods. However, the afterload estimated by the systolic blood pressure/heart rate product did not change significantly after nifedipine.[27,28,42] It may be concluded that there is some effect with afterload reduction or vasodilator therapy. However, it should be noted that these results lack large study populations or hard outcomes data. Thus, large-scale evidence-based therapy has not been established.

Ventricular Systolic Dysfunction

Systolic or diastolic dysfunction may occur early in SSc heart disease, years before becoming clinically evident.[21,22] This finding is particularly true in the case of patients with SSc with left ventricular diastolic dysfunction, whereas systolic dysfunction is less common and occurs mainly because of concomitant coronary artery disease or hypertensive heart disease.[21,43] Systolic dysfunction is much less common than diastolic dysfunction, with recent studies reporting an incidence between 11% and 15%.[44]

Radionuclide ventriculography has been used to assess LVEF and right ventricular ejection fraction (RVEF) and peak filling rate.[19,45–47] Several studies reported a decreased global LVEF in a minority of patients, although segmental dysfunction or exercise-induced dysfunction was more prevalent.[48,49] In one study of 26 patients with dcSSc, 4 had reduced LVEF and 7 had reduced RVEF, including the 4 patients with reduced LVEF.[45] In another study, 42 consecutive patients with SSc with normal pulmonary arterial pressure and less than 5 years of disease duration were compared with 20 matched controls.[50] Sixteen patients had reduced RVEF, 3 had reduced LVEF, and 10 had reduced peak filling rate (an indicator of early right systolic and left diastolic dysfunction). RVEF correlated with LVEF and the peak filling rate, whereas no correlation was found with either pulmonary function impairment or pulmonary arterial pressure, implying intrinsic myocardial involvement in these patients rather than a secondary effect.

The association of myocardial perfusion abnormalities with myocardial dysfunction suggests a common mechanism for myocardial involvement. Myocardial perfusion, as examined by thallium perfusion scans, is likely a marker of microvascular ischemia. Thallium perfusion defect scores more than the median were associated with a significantly lower mean LVEF, and all patients with abnormal resting LVEF had thallium scores more than the median. Nicardipine was shown to acutely improve global LVEF and segmental abnormalities and to improve LVEF and RVEF.[48,50] These results provide further evidence for a similar pathogenic pathway with reversible vasospastic small coronary artery disease inducing segmental and global heart dysfunction.

Allanore and colleagues[51] evaluated 129 patients with SSc and LVEF less than 55% compared with 256 patients with SSc with normal LVEF. They demonstrated that male sex, age, digital ulcerations, myositis, and lack of treatment with calcium-channel blockers were independent factors associated with left ventricular dysfunction. However, typical cardiovascular risk factors were not associated with reduced LVEF, suggesting that indicators of severity of SSc as well as markers of microvascular lesions, such as digital ulcerations, are associated with reduced LVEF.

There are no long-term outcome studies of the treatment of systolic dysfunction associated with scleroderma. Traditional therapy for heart failure is implemented, including diuretics, angiotensin-converting enzyme inhibitors (or angiotensin-receptor blockers), and aldosterone antagonists. Calcium-channel blockers may also be used because the pathophysiology for systolic dysfunction is similar to that of diastolic dysfunction.

Myositis and Myocarditis

Inflammatory myocarditis has been recognized as a possible complication of scleroderma and is usually associated with skeletal muscle myositis. Cardiac MRI allows for the identification of myocarditis and may assist in the morphologic evaluation of affected myocardium compared with viable tissue.[52] Serum creatinine kinase MB isoenzyme elevation in conjunction with echocardiography has also been used to diagnose and monitor myocarditis.[53]

PERICARDIAL DISEASE

There is a wide spectrum of pericardial involvement in SSc, which includes acute pericarditis, chronic pericarditis, pericardial fibrosis, and pericardial effusion. Pericardial effusion is rarely complicated by cardiac tamponade. Although pericardial involvement is often asymptomatic, some patients may experience a wide range of symptoms. The incidence of pericardial involvement varies from 33% to 72%, but symptomatic disease is estimated to be only 7% to 20%.[54]

Acute and Chronic Pericarditis

Acute, symptomatic pericarditis is an uncommon manifestation of SSc. Case reports of acute pericarditis and pericardial effusion are well described, but a significant amount of data regarding pericardial disease has been developed from study at autopsy (consequently with little history available). Patients with SSc and renal disease may have uremic pericarditis or pericardial effusion, clouding the relationship between SSc and pericardial disease. Acute pericarditis classically presents with symptoms of positional retrosternal chest pain that is pleuritic in nature. Acute pericarditis is associated with ECG findings of diffuse ST-segment elevation and typically responds well to treatment with nonsteroidal antiinflammatory drug (NSAID) therapy. Concurrent symptoms and signs may include fever, dyspnea, pericardial friction rub, or referred scapular pain. Colchicine, with standard doses of 1 mg/day (or up to 2 mg/day for loading doses), has been validated in a prospective study as a monotherapy or in conjunction with aspirin.[55] The duration of therapy should be 1 to 3 months, depending on the intensity of disease. Acute pericarditis may be associated with pericardial effusion, which may or may not resolve with time. Large pericardial effusion should be recognized as a risk factor for the development of scleroderma renal crisis.[7] As with other causes of pericarditis, the treatment of SSc-associated pericarditis with corticosteroids is not advised because of an increased risk of transformation to chronic symptomatic pericarditis. Steroid therapy at moderate to high doses is also a known precipitant of scleroderma renal crisis.

Chronic or recurrent pericarditis may present with relapsing, intermittent symptoms, or incessant disease that flares whenever therapy is withheld. Relapsing pericarditis may have widely varying asymptomatic periods. Viral or bacterial infections and other reversible causes should be excluded as an explanation for recurrent disease, which may be accomplished through the analysis of pericardial fluid or tissue obtained from pericardiocentesis or biopsy. Corticosteroids should only be used in refractory cases with frequent crises unresponsive to NSAID therapy and colchicine. If steroids are indicated, dosing options include oral therapy, most commonly with prednisone, or intrapericardial triamcinolone injection. The European Society of Cardiology's guidelines recommend prednisone at 1.0 to 1.5 mg/kg for at least 1 month, with concurrent use of gastrointestinal protective therapy.[56] However, prednisone therapy in dosages greater than 15 mg/d increases the risk of scleroderma renal crisis. When beginning steroid tapering, it is recommended to restart colchicine with or without an NSAID. Additionally, azathioprine or cyclophosphamide may be used as adjunctive therapy for patients who do not respond to corticosteroids.

CONDUCTION DISEASE AND DYSRHYTHMIAS

A wide spectrum of conduction system disease and dysrhythmias is diagnosed in patients with SSc. Myocardial fibrosis and autonomic cardiac neuropathy are thought to underlie the predisposition to supraventricular and ventricular dysrhythmias, which could be responsible for sudden death in some individuals.[38,39,48,57] Resting ECG remains an important screening tool used for the identification of electrical system disease in patients with SSc. In a series of 436 patients with SSc, 25% had an abnormal ECG; PR segment prolongation, left anterior fascicular block, and intraventricular conduction defects were the most common findings. The prevalence of conduction disturbances is significantly higher on 24-hour ambulatory ECG (Holter) monitoring compared with resting ECG.[58,59]

Supraventricular tachycardias are the most frequent finding on Holter monitoring. Ventricular dysrhythmias, including multiform or coupled ventricular premature contractions and runs of ventricular tachycardia, are less common.[58,59] Importantly, ventricular dysrhythmias are correlated with an increased risk of sudden death and mortality.[19,24] Patients with ventricular dysrhythmias and concurrent skeletal muscle involvement have a worse prognosis compared with other patients with ventricular dysrhythmias.[49] In the aforementioned series, the incidence of cardiac dysrhythmias seems to have decreased over the last 2 decades. It is hypothesized that patient screening has led to earlier intervention. Additionally, newer therapies, including those for pulmonary hypertension, have lessened the likelihood of developing dysrhythmia.

Various investigators using conventional testing methods have reported autonomic neuropathy in SSc.[19,24,60] Dysfunction in the autonomic control of heart rate activity may contribute to dysrhythmias and to the severity of scleroderma heart disease. Computerized analysis of the heart rate variability by means of 24-hour Holter monitoring has been proposed as a noninvasive tool to screen for autonomic abnormalities.[61] This study demonstrated a significantly higher heart rate and lower circadian and spectral indexes of heart rate variability in patients with SSc compared with control subjects. The findings of tachycardia, low circadian heart rate variability, and spectral power values predicted higher mortality. Autonomic cardiac neuropathy may represent an important prognostic feature that should be considered in evaluation of all patients with SSc with, at minimum, baseline ECG and monitoring of symptoms.

Case studies and small case series have described advanced conduction disease or heart block in SSc, which is thought to be a rare problem. There is minimal information regarding the need for pacemaker implantation; the indications for pacemaker implantation should be determined using traditional criteria as applicable to the general population.

VASCULAR DISEASE AND LESS COMMON MANIFESTATIONS

Vascular disease associated with SSc predominantly affects the small arteries and arterioles rather than major epicardial coronary arteries. The histologic study of the intramural coronaries has revealed concentric intimal hyperplasia associated with fibrinoid necrosis.[8] Patients with intramural coronary artery involvement may experience angina and myocardial infarction in the absence of significant epicardial coronary artery disease. The frequency of obstructive atherosclerotic disease of the large coronary arteries seems to be similar to that of the general population.[57] In contrast, one recent autopsy study found significantly more atherosclerosis in patients with SSc than in controls.[33,62] Although the presence of medium-sized vessel coronary atherosclerosis was similar (48% vs 43%), atherosclerotic lesions of small coronary arteries or arterioles were found in 17% of the patients with SSc and only 2% of the controls.

Early coronary dysfunction can be identified as a reduction in coronary flow reserve (CFR). A low CFR is associated with an increased risk of major cardiac events. CFR is lower in patients with SSc compared with age- and gender-matched controls.[62] Coronary flow reserve at left heart catheterization has been investigated in patients with dcSSc.[63] As a measure of coronary flow, mean coronary sinus blood flow was not significantly different at rest in patients with SSc compared with control subjects. After maximal coronary vasodilation with intravenous dipyridamole, flow reserve was strikingly reduced in patients with scleroderma. Coronary angiograms were normal, but fibrotic tissue with concentric intimal hyperplasia of intramural coronary arteries and arterioles was observed on endomyocardial biopsy specimens. Therefore, it is postulated that pathologic changes in small coronary arteries and arterioles explains the reduced coronary reserve. These arterial changes likely predispose the myocardium to ischemia related to myocardial Raynaud phenomenon. Despite a demonstration of impaired coronary flow, a causal relationship between impaired coronary flow and myocardial fibrosis has not been definitively elucidated. Recent studies using contrast-enhanced transthoracic Doppler echocardiography before and after adenosine infusion have shown impaired CFR in the absence of clinical myocardial involvement.[38,64]

Other noninvasive testing may help identify patients at risk for significant atherosclerosis. Calcium scoring by computed tomography scans may demonstrate at least moderate to severe coronary calcifications in up to two-thirds of patients with SSc.[65] Ultrasonography to evaluate carotid intima media thickness in patients with SSc has been found to be useful in diagnosing subclinical systemic atherosclerosis.[62] Because carotid atherosclerosis is a predictor of subsequent myocardial infarction and stroke, the identification of underlying atherosclerotic disease is important for intervention before progression of disease.

Vasospasm of the small coronary arteries or arterioles plays a major role in the early myocardial abnormalities in SSc. Repeated ischemia reperfusion abnormalities may be the cause of irreversible myocardial fibrosis. The presence of myocardial Raynaud phenomenon has been debated. Investigation of this theory has been attempted with thallium-201 SPECT to assess for myocardial perfusion abnormalities. Multiple studies have demonstrated that coronary vasospasm induced by cold-pressor testing is observed much more frequently in patients with SSc compared with controls, even among asymptomatic patients.[39,57,66] The increased incidence of coronary vasospasm suggests a functional Raynaud phenomenon of the heart. To test this theory, various studies have investigated vasodilator therapy, including dipyridamole, nifedipine, nicardipine, and captopril. SPECT imaging and thallium perfusion scans showed improved perfusion in all cases after vasodilator therapy.[32,46,47,67] However, a clinical benefit has not been well established. Using stress thallium-201 myocardial SPECT, decreased perfusion was observed in 82% of all patients with SSc studied. The incidence of fixed defects, reversible defects, or reverse redistribution was significantly higher in symptomatic patients with SSc.[68] The coexistence of both reversible and fixed defects, often in the same patient, suggests that arteriolar vasospasm may potentially coexist with fixed coronary lesions.

Positron emission tomography studies have demonstrated the beneficial effect of nifedipine on myocardial perfusion and metabolism in patients with SSc. In one study, there was a significant increase in 38 K myocardial uptake and a significant decrease in 18 fludeoxyglucose uptake indicating improvement in both myocardial perfusion and metabolism.[69] It is hypothesized that coronary arteriolar vasospasm might be more relevant in an early, perhaps preclinical phase of myocardial involvement, whereas increased collagen deposition becomes predominant with disease progression.

More recently, cardiovascular MRI has been lauded as an accurate, quantitative method for the noninvasive assessment of myocardial perfusion.[70] High-resolution perfusion MRI techniques may be used to identify small subendocardial perfusion defects, such as those thought to be related to microvascular ischemia in SSc. Using MRI in patients with SSc, treatment with nifedipine (before and after 14 days of 60 mg/d) was shown to provide an average 38% increase of the global perfusion index and a decrease in the number of patients with more than one segmental perfusion defect, from 7 out of 18 (39%) to zero out of 18 ($P<.05$).[42]

Significant valvular disease is not common in SSc, and data from echocardiography studies and specimens at autopsy have shown a low incidence of major valvular lesions.[18] Nodular thickening of the mitral and aortic valves is the most common abnormality described and may intermittently be associated with valvular regurgitation.[71–73]

DIAGNOSTIC EVALUATION

The diagnostic evaluation for cardiac involvement in scleroderma patients requires a careful history and physical examination in addition to basic testing (**Fig. 2**). Symptoms such as dyspnea, decreased exercise tolerance, fatigue, and chest discomfort, though nonspecific and possibly multifactorial, are most often reported by patients with SSc and cardiac and/or pulmonary involvement.[24]

The severity of dyspnea is measured according to established New York Heart Association's guidelines. Although subjective, this classification assists in achieving objective quantification of functional limitation with different stress testing protocols. Physical examination should include both auscultation and palpation of the heart. The presence or absence of rales, murmurs, dysrhythmia, jugular venous distention, hepatomegaly, and lower-extremity edema provides diagnostic and prognostic information.

First-line noninvasive diagnostic tests include ECG, chest radiograph, and Doppler echocardiography. The ECG quickly provides information on conduction system function and indirectly evaluates the autonomic control of sinus node function. Atrial and ventricular enlargement, vascular congestion, interstitial lung disease, and pleuropericardial abnormalities can be detected on chest radiographs. The Doppler-echocardiogram can assess for the presence of pericardial effusion, left ventricular systolic and diastolic dysfunction, right ventricular impairment, and atrial or ventricular volumes. Echocardiography can also indirectly evaluate the presence and magnitude of pulmonary hypertension.

A 6-minute walk test or exercise bicycle/treadmill stress test may be useful in providing information regarding conditioning and cardiac performance, particularly if the history is unclear. One caveat when assessing arterial oxygen saturation during exercise (eg, 6-minute walk test) is the unreliability of a fingertip oximeter in patients with SSc who nearly always have Raynaud phenomenon and digital ischemia; oximeter

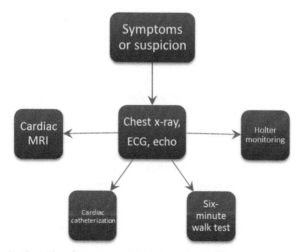

Fig. 2. Diagnostic algorithm for potential heart disease in SSc.

readings from the forehead seem to be much more reliable when assessing patients with SSc. Formal cardiopulmonary exercise testing may be beneficial to further quantify performance capabilities. Placement of arterial lines should be avoided in patients with SSc. Depending on the need for further testing, a variety of diagnostic studies are available, including ambulatory Holter monitoring; nuclear myocardial perfusion scintigraphy; echocardiography with assessment of coronary flow reserve; cardiac MRI; ultrasonic video densitometric analysis (to detect preclinical alterations suggestive of myocardial fibrosis); and finally, right heart cardiac catheterization (potentially with vasodilatory drug study).

FUTURE DIRECTIONS AND SUMMARY

Although definitive therapy for heart disease related to SSc has been elusive, novel approaches are being explored. Although still considered to be investigational and of uncertain efficacy, hematopoietic stem cell transplantation (HSCT) is being offered to an increasing number of patients with SSc. Burt and colleagues[74] recently reported results from their 2-center experience, citing a 6% treatment-related mortality after HSCT and a significant improvement in skin disease and pulmonary forced vital capacity. Despite routine pretransplant echocardiography, 4 of the 5 reported deaths in this study resulted from cardiac-related causes. The investigators concluded that guidelines for cardiac screening of patients with SSc to assess the treatment-related risk from pulmonary arterial hypertension, primary cardiac involvement, or pericardial disease should be reconsidered and potentially intensified. It is hoped that HSCT might demonstrate improvement in heart disease related to SSc, but this has not been investigated to date. Cyclophosphamide and imatinib are other potential therapies for patients with SSc, but data regarding efficacy in heart disease associated with SSc are also lacking.

The cardiac disease associated with scleroderma can present in many forms and is often clinically silent until significant organ dysfunction has ensued. As clinical awareness and diagnostic methods have improved, earlier detection and treatment are both feasible and advisable. Awareness of heart disease associated with SSc, whether clinically evident or occult, is now an important part of the management.

REFERENCES

1. Goetz RH, Berne MB. The pathology of progressive systemic sclerosis (generalized scleroderma) with special reference to changes in viscera. Mayo Clin Proc 1945;4:337.
2. Rodnan GP, Benedek TG. An historical account of the study of progressive systemic sclerosis (diffuse scleroderma). Ann Intern Med 1962;57:305–19.
3. Heine J. Uber ein eigenartiges Krankheitsbild von deiffuser Sklerosis der haut and innerer organe. Virchows Arch A Pathol Anat Histol 1926;262(1):1562–89.
4. Weiss SE, Warren J. Scleroderma heart disease, with a consideration of certain other visceral manifestations of cardiopulmonary disease in progressive systemic sclerosis. Arch Intern Med 1943;71:749–76.
5. Weiss SE, Warren J. Scleroderma heart disease, with a consideration of certain other visceral manifestations of scleroderma. Arch Intern Med 1943;71:1.
6. Bulkley BH, Ridolfi RL, Salyer WR, et al. Myocardial lesions of progressive systemic sclerosis. A cause of cardiac dysfunction. Circulation 1976;53(3):483–90.
7. McWhorter JE, LeRoy EC. Pericardial disease in scleroderma (systemic sclerosis). Am J Med 1974;57(4):566–75.

8. James TN. De subitaneis mortibus. VIII. Coronary arteries and conduction system in scleroderma heart disease. Circulation 1974;50(4):844–56.
9. Kahan A, Coghlan G, McLaughlin V. Cardiac complications of systemic sclerosis. Rheumatology (Oxford) 2009;48(Suppl 3):iii45–8.
10. Medsger TA Jr, Masi AT. Survival with scleroderma. II. A life-table analysis of clinical and demographic factors in 358 male U.S. veteran patients. J Chronic Dis 1973;26(10):647–60.
11. Steen VD, Medsger TA Jr. Severe organ involvement in systemic sclerosis with diffuse scleroderma. Arthritis Rheum 2000;43(11):2437–44.
12. Ferri C, Valentini G, Cozzi F, et al. Systemic sclerosis: demographic, clinical, and serologic features and survival in 1,012 Italian patients. Medicine (Baltimore) 2002;81(2):139–53.
13. Elhai M, Meune C, Avouac J, et al. Trends in mortality in patients with systemic sclerosis over 40 years: a systematic review and meta-analysis of cohort studies. Rheumatology (Oxford) 2012;51(6):1017–26.
14. Domsic RT, Rodriguez-Reyna T, Lucas M, et al. Skin thickness progression rate: a predictor of mortality and early internal organ involvement in diffuse scleroderma. Ann Rheum Dis 2011;70(1):104–9.
15. Hachulla AL, Launay D, Gaxotte V, et al. Cardiac magnetic resonance imaging in systemic sclerosis: a cross-sectional observational study of 52 patients. Ann Rheum Dis 2009;68(12):1878–84.
16. de Groote P, Gressin V, Hachulla E, et al. Evaluation of cardiac abnormalities by Doppler echocardiography in a large nationwide multicentric cohort of patients with systemic sclerosis. Ann Rheum Dis 2008;67(1):31–6.
17. Steen VD, Powell DL, Medsger TA Jr. Clinical correlations and prognosis based on serum autoantibodies in patients with systemic sclerosis. Arthritis Rheum 1988;31(2):196–203.
18. Medsger TA. Systemic sclerosis (scleroderma): clinical aspects. In: Koopman WJ, editor. Arthritis and allied conditions. Philadelphia: Lippincott Williams & Wikins; 2001.
19. Deswal A, Follansbee WP. Cardiac involvement in scleroderma. Rheum Dis Clin North Am 1996;22(4):841–60.
20. D'Angelo WA, Fries JF, Masi AT, et al. Pathologic observations in systemic sclerosis (scleroderma). A study of fifty-eight autopsy cases and fifty-eight matched controls. Am J Med 1969;46(3):428–40.
21. Armstrong GP, Whalley GA, Doughty RN, et al. Left ventricular function in scleroderma. Br J Rheumatol 1996;35(10):983–8.
22. Valentini G, Vitale DF, Giunta A, et al. Diastolic abnormalities in systemic sclerosis: evidence for associated defective cardiac functional reserve. Ann Rheum Dis 1996;55(7):455–60.
23. Aguglia G, Sgreccia A, Bernardo ML, et al. Left ventricular diastolic function in systemic sclerosis. J Rheumatol 2001;28(7):1563–7.
24. Ferri C, Emdin M, Nielsen H, et al. Assessment of heart involvement. Clin Exp Rheumatol 2003;21(3 Suppl 29):S24–8.
25. Giunta A, Tirri E, Maione S, et al. Right ventricular diastolic abnormalities in systemic sclerosis. Relation to left ventricular involvement and pulmonary hypertension. Ann Rheum Dis 2000;59(2):94–8.
26. Uematsu M, Nakatani S, Yamagishi M, et al. Usefulness of myocardial velocity gradient derived from two-dimensional tissue Doppler imaging as an indicator of regional myocardial contraction independent of translational motion assessed in atrial septal defect. Am J Cardiol 1997;79(2):237–41.

27. Derumeaux G, Mulder P, Richard V, et al. Tissue Doppler imaging differentiates physiological from pathological pressure-overload left ventricular hypertrophy in rats. Circulation 2002;105(13):1602–8.

28. Smiseth OA, Ihlen H. Strain rate imaging: why do we need it? J Am Coll Cardiol 2003;42(9):1584–6.

29. Meune C, Pascal O, Bécane HM, et al. Reliable detection of early myocardial dysfunction by tissue Doppler echocardiography in Becker muscular dystrophy. Heart 2004;90(8):947–8.

30. Plazak W, Zabinska-Plazak E, Wojas-Pelc A, et al. Heart structure and function in systemic sclerosis. Eur J Dermatol 2002;12(3):257–62.

31. Scussel-Lonzetti L, Joyal F, Raynauld JP, et al. Predicting mortality in systemic sclerosis: analysis of a cohort of 309 French Canadian patients with emphasis on features at diagnosis as predictive factors for survival. Medicine (Baltimore) 2002;81(2):154–67.

32. Kahan A, Devaux JY, Amor B, et al. Pharmacodynamic effect of dipyridamole on thallium-201 myocardial perfusion in progressive systemic sclerosis with diffuse scleroderma. Ann Rheum Dis 1986;45(9):718–25.

33. Kahan A, Allanore Y. Primary myocardial involvement in systemic sclerosis. Rheumatology (Oxford) 2006;45(Suppl 4):iv14–7.

34. Nakajima K, Taki J, Kawano M, et al. Diastolic dysfunction in patients with systemic sclerosis detected by gated myocardial perfusion SPECT: an early sign of cardiac involvement. J Nucl Med 2001;42(2):183–8.

35. Boueiz A, Mathai SC, Hummers LK, et al. Cardiac complications of systemic sclerosis: recent progress in diagnosis. Curr Opin Rheumatol 2010;22(6): 696–703.

36. Tzelepis GE, Kelekis NL, Plastiras SC, et al. Pattern and distribution of myocardial fibrosis in systemic sclerosis: a delayed enhanced magnetic resonance imaging study. Arthritis Rheum 2007;56(11):3827–36.

37. Meune C, Allanore Y, Pascal O, et al. Myocardial contractility is early affected in systemic sclerosis: a tissue Doppler echocardiography study. Eur J Echocardiogr 2005;6(5):351–7.

38. Sulli A, Ghio M, Bezante GP, et al. Blunted coronary flow reserve in systemic sclerosis. Rheumatology (Oxford) 2004;43(4):505–9.

39. Gustafsson R, Mannting F, Kazzam E, et al. Cold-induced reversible myocardial ischaemia in systemic sclerosis. Lancet 1989;2(8661):475–9.

40. Bilan A, Chibowska M, Makaruk B, et al. Enalapril (10 mg/day) in systemic sclerosis. One year, double blind, randomised study (ESS-1): echocardiographic substudy–three months follow-up. Adv Exp Med Biol 1999;455:279–83.

41. Kazzam E, Caidahl K, HIlgren R, et al. Non-invasive evaluation of long-term cardiac effects of captopril in systemic sclerosis. J Intern Med 1991;230(3):203–12.

42. Vignaux O, Allanore Y, Meune C, et al. Evaluation of the effect of nifedipine upon myocardial perfusion and contractility using cardiac magnetic resonance imaging and tissue Doppler echocardiography in systemic sclerosis. Ann Rheum Dis 2005;64(9):1268–73.

43. Maione S, Cuomo G, Giunta A, et al. Echocardiographic alterations in systemic sclerosis: a longitudinal study. Semin Arthritis Rheum 2005;34(5):721–7.

44. Champion HC. The heart in scleroderma. Rheum Dis Clin North Am 2008;34(1): 181–90, viii.

45. Follansbee WP, Curtiss EI, Medsger TA Jr, et al. Physiologic abnormalities of cardiac function in progressive systemic sclerosis with diffuse scleroderma. N Engl J Med 1984;310(3):142–8.

46. Kahan A, Devaux JY, Amor B, et al. Nicardipine improves myocardial perfusion in systemic sclerosis. J Rheumatol 1988;15(9):1395–400.
47. Kahan A, et al. Nifedipine and thallium-201 myocardial perfusion in progressive systemic sclerosis. N Engl J Med 1986;314(22):1397–402.
48. Kahan A, Devaux JY, Amor B, et al. Pharmacodynamic effect of nicardipine on left ventricular function in systemic sclerosis. J Cardiovasc Pharmacol 1990; 15(2):249–53.
49. Follansbee WP, Zerbe TR, Medsger TA Jr. Cardiac and skeletal muscle disease in systemic sclerosis (scleroderma): a high risk association. Am Heart J 1993; 125(1):194–203.
50. Meune C, Allanore Y, Devaux JY, et al. High prevalence of right ventricular systolic dysfunction in early systemic sclerosis. J Rheumatol 2004;31(10):1941–5.
51. Allanore Y, Meune C, Vonk MC, et al. Prevalence and factors associated with left ventricular dysfunction in the EULAR Scleroderma Trial and Research group (EUSTAR) database of patients with systemic sclerosis. Ann Rheum Dis 2010; 69(1):218–21.
52. Allanore Y, Vignaux O, Arnaud L, et al. Effects of corticosteroids and immunosuppressors on idiopathic inflammatory myopathy related myocarditis evaluated by magnetic resonance imaging. Ann Rheum Dis 2006;65(2):249–52.
53. Kerr LD, Spiera H. Myocarditis as a complication in scleroderma patients with myositis. Clin Cardiol 1993;16(12):895–9.
54. Byers RJ, Marshall DA, Freemont AJ. Pericardial involvement in systemic sclerosis. Ann Rheum Dis 1997;56(6):393–4.
55. Imazio M, Bobbio M, Cecchi E, et al. Colchicine in addition to conventional therapy for acute pericarditis: results of the COlchicine for acute PEricarditis (COPE) trial. Circulation 2005;112(13):2012–6.
56. Maisch B, Seferović PM, Ristić AD, et al. Guidelines on the diagnosis and management of pericardial diseases executive summary; the task force on the diagnosis and management of pericardial diseases of the European Society of Cardiology. Eur Heart J 2004;25(7):587–610.
57. Candell-Riera J, Armadans-Gil L, Simeón CP, et al. Comprehensive noninvasive assessment of cardiac involvement in limited systemic sclerosis. Arthritis Rheum 1996;39(7):1138–45.
58. Ferri C, Bernini L, Bongiorni MG, et al. Noninvasive evaluation of cardiac dysrhythmias, and their relationship with multisystemic symptoms, in progressive systemic sclerosis patients. Arthritis Rheum 1985;28(11):1259–66.
59. Roberts NK, Cabeen WR Jr, Moss J, et al. The prevalence of conduction defects and cardiac arrhythmias in progressive systemic sclerosis. Ann Intern Med 1981;94(1):38–40.
60. Dessein PH, Joffe BI, Metz RM, et al. Autonomic dysfunction in systemic sclerosis: sympathetic overactivity and instability. Am J Med 1992;93(2):143–50.
61. Ferri C, Emdin M, Giuggioli D, et al. Autonomic dysfunction in systemic sclerosis: time and frequency domain 24 hour heart rate variability analysis. Br J Rheumatol 1997;36(6):669–76.
62. Kaloudi O, Matucci Cerinic M. Systemic sclerosis: the heart puzzle. Rheumatologist 2009;3(13):5. Available at: http://www.the-rheumatologist.org/details/article/872231/The_Heart-SCC_Puzzle.html.
63. Kahan A, Nitenberg A, Foult JM, et al. Decreased coronary reserve in primary scleroderma myocardial disease. Arthritis Rheum 1985;28(6):637–46.
64. Montisci R, Vacca A, Garau P, et al. Detection of early impairment of coronary flow reserve in patients with systemic sclerosis. Ann Rheum Dis 2003;62(9):890–3.

65. Mok MY, Lau CS, Chiu SS, et al. Systemic sclerosis is an independent risk factor for increased coronary artery calcium deposition. Arthritis Rheum 2011;63(5): 1387–95.
66. Alexander EL, Firestein GS, Weiss JL, et al. Reversible cold-induced abnormalities in myocardial perfusion and function in systemic sclerosis. Ann Intern Med 1986;105(5):661–8.
67. Kahan A, Devaux JY, Amor B, et al. The effect of captopril on thallium 201 myocardial perfusion in systemic sclerosis. Clin Pharmacol Ther 1990;47(4): 483–9.
68. Ishida R, Murata Y, Sawada Y, et al. Thallium-201 myocardial SPET in patients with collagen disease. Nucl Med Commun 2000;21(8):729–34.
69. Duboc D, Kahan A, Maziere B, et al. The effect of nifedipine on myocardial perfusion and metabolism in systemic sclerosis. A positron emission tomographic study. Arthritis Rheum 1991;34(2):198–203.
70. Nagel E, Klein C, Paetsch I, et al. Magnetic resonance perfusion measurements for the noninvasive detection of coronary artery disease. Circulation 2003; 108(4):432–7.
71. Gottdiener JS, Moutsopoulos HM, Decker JL. Echocardiographic identification of cardiac abnormality in scleroderma and related disorders. Am J Med 1979; 66(3):391–8.
72. Kinney E, Reeves W, Zellis R. The echocardiogram in scleroderma endocarditis of the mitral valve. Arch Intern Med 1979;139(10):1179–80.
73. Smith JW, Clements PJ, Levisman J, et al. Echocardiographic features of progressive systemic sclerosis (PSS). Correlation with hemodynamic and postmortem studies. Am J Med 1979;66(1):28–33.
74. Burt RK, Oliveira MC, Shah SJ, et al. Cardiac involvement and treatment-related mortality after non-myeloablative haemopoietic stem-cell transplantation with unselected autologous peripheral blood for patients with systemic sclerosis: a retrospective analysis. Lancet 2013;381(9872):1116–24.

Pulmonary Arterial Hypertension Related to Connective Tissue Disease: A Review

Saman Ahmed, MD[a],*, Harold I. Palevsky, MD[b]

KEYWORDS

- Pulmonary arterial hypertension • Associated pulmonary arterial hypertension
- Connective tissue disease related PAH • PAH and scleroderma
- PAH and systemic lupus erythematosus
- Transthoracic echocardiogram in pulmonary arterial hypertension

KEY POINTS

- Pulmonary hypertension (PH) is defined as mean pulmonary artery pressure (mPAP) greater than or equal to 25 mm Hg in a resting condition as measured by right heart catheterization.
- Pulmonary arterial hypertension (PAH) is defined as an mPAP greater than or equal to 25 mm Hg in the setting of normal left atrial pressures (usually measured as the pulmonary capillary wedge pressure (PCWP) less than or equal to 15 mm Hg).
- Connective tissue disease (CTD)-related PAH falls within the category of associated pulmonary arterial hypertension (APAH) within Group I of the current classification of PH.
- The incidence of APAH in CTD varies with CTD etiology, and can be as high as 60% in mixed connective tissue disease (MCTD).
- These disorders have a significant morbidity and a high mortality, thus an early diagnosis and treatment is essential for improving the outcomes.

INTRODUCTION AND DEFINITION

Pulmonary hypertension (PH) is an increase in pulmonary artery pressure in the pulmonary vascular bed that ultimately may lead to progressive right heart strain and

Funding Resources: None.
Conflict of Interest: S. Ahmed, None; H. Palevsky has served as a consultant to Acelion Pharmaceuticals, Aires Pharmaceuticals, Bayer HealthCare and United Therapeutics.
a Medical Intensive Care Unit, Department of Medicine, Penn Presbyterian Medical Center, University of Pennsylvania Health System, 51 North 39th Street, Cupp Building, Philadelphia, PA 19104-2699, USA; b Pulmonary Vascular Disease Program, Penn Presbyterian Medical Center, Perelman School of Medicine, University of Pennsylvania, 51 North 39th Street, Suite 120, PHI Building, Philadelphia, PA 19104-2699, USA
* Corresponding author.
E-mail address: Saman.Ahmed@uphs.upenn.edu

Rheum Dis Clin N Am 40 (2014) 103–124
http://dx.doi.org/10.1016/j.rdc.2013.10.001
0889-857X/14/$ – see front matter © 2014 Elsevier Inc. All rights reserved.

ultimately, right heart failure.[1,2] It is defined as a mean pulmonary artery pressure (mPAP) greater than or equal to 25 mm Hg in resting condition as measured by right heart catheterization.[3,4] Pulmonary arterial hypertension (PAH) is a subgroup of PH, which is defined as increase in mPAP of greater than or equal to 25 mm Hg with a normal left atrial pressure (most often assessed as a pulmonary capillary wedge pressure [PCWP] of less than or equal to 15 mm Hg) and a normal or reduced cardiac output in the absence of intrinsic lung disease or chronic unresolved pulmonary emboli (**Table 1**).[2,4] Expanded criteria for defining PAH in patients being evaluated in the Registry to EValuate EArly and Long term pulmonary arterial hypertension management (REVEAL Registry) defines PAH as has been done previously, but is also evaluating the impact of including patients with a PCWP of 16 to 18 mm Hg within the definition.[5] A previously proposed definition of PH during exercise (ie, mPAP greater than or equal to 30 mm Hg with exercise) is no longer being used, as there are no data supporting a single number to define the upper limit of normal mPAP during exercise[6]; factors such as age, type of exercise, and exercise workload appear to determine the normal response of PA pressures with exercise.[7]

CLASSIFICATION OF PH

An initial classification of PH was published in 1973 following the First World Symposium on Pulmonary Hypertension, and divided the PH into 2 broad categories of primary and secondary PH.[8] In 1998, the Second World Symposium on Pulmonary Hypertension revised the classification and divided PH in to 5 broad categories: (1) PAH, (2) pulmonary venous hypertension, (3) PH associated with disorders of the respiratory system or hypoxemia, (4) PH caused by thrombotic or embolic diseases, and (5) PH caused by diseases affecting the pulmonary vasculature.[9–11] This classification was subsequently modified in the third and fourth World Symposia on PH in 2003 and 2008 respectively.[8,12–14] The most recent modifications (adopted in 2008) were to Groups I, IV, V; however, the basic architecture of the PH classification was maintained.[8,15,16] Group I PH is PAH and includes idiopathic PAH (IPAH), heritable PAH (HPAH), drug-induced and toxin-induced PAH, and associated PAH (APAH). Connective tissue disease (CTD)-related PAH falls within the category of APAH in Group I. A complete detailing of the current classification is presented in **Table 1**.

PATHOGENESIS

The pulmonary circulation is normally a high-flow, low-resistance vascular bed that is in series with the systemic circulation and accommodates the entire cardiac output through one organ.[17] The flow in this system is normally regulated by multiple factors, including oxygen and carbon dioxide tensions, the sympathetic nervous system, and hormonal stimuli.[17] These factors result in either vasoconstriction or vasodilatation of the precapillary pulmonary vasculature, which alters the pulmonary vascular resistance and effects cardiac output and pulmonary arterial pressures. Alveolar hypoxia is one of the main stimuli that cause pulmonary arterial vasoconstriction, either directly or indirectly by contributing to the release of mediators.[17,18] Several mediators impacting the pulmonary arterial vascular bed, including endothelin-1 (ET-1), nitric oxide (NO), prostacyclin, angiopoietin-1, serotonin, and members of the transforming-growth-factor-beta superfamily, have been identified, and serve as targets for therapeutic agents (available and investigational) for PH.[19]

ET-1 is a potent endothelium-derived vasoconstrictor that also appears to be involved in remodeling of the pulmonary vasculature by initiating mitosis of pulmonary vascular smooth muscle cells and fibroblasts.[20] It also acts to constrict the

Table 1
Clinical classification of pulmonary hypertension

Group 1: Pulmonary Arterial Hypertension	Group 1: PAH Associated with Venous/Capillary Involvement	Group 2: PH Related to Left Heart Failure	Group 3: PH Related to Lung Diseases and/or Hypoxia	Group 4: Chronic Thromboembolic PH	Group 5: PH due to Unclear or Multifactorial Mechanisms
1. Idiopathic (IPAH) 2. Heritable (includes BMPR2, ALK1, endogolin with or without hemorrhagic telangiectasia and unknown) 3. Drugs and toxin induced (fenfluramine, dexfenfluramine, amphetamine, aminorex, toxic rapeseed oil, L-tryptophan, methamphetamines) 4. Associated (APAH) (includes CTD, HIV, congenital heart disease, schistosomiasis, and chronic hemolytic anemia)	1. Pulmonary veno-occlusive disease 2. Pulmonary capillary hemangiomatosis	1. Systolic dysfunction 2. Diastolic dysfunction 3. Valvular disease	1. COPD 2. ILD 3. Mixed restrictive and obstructive diseases 4. Sleep-disordered breathing 5. Alveolar hypoventilation disorder 6. Chronic high altitude exposure 7. Developmental abnormalities	1. Chronic thromboembolic disease	1. Hematologic disorders, such as myeloproliferative diseases, splenectomy 2. Systemic disorders, such as sarcoidosis, langerhan histiocytosis, lymphangioleiomyomatosis, neurofibromatosis, vasculitis 3. Metabolic disorders, such as Gaucher disease, glycogen storage diseases, thyroid disorders 4. Others include chronic renal failure on dialysis, tumoral obstruction, fibrosing mediastinitis

Abbreviations: CTD, connective tissue disease; PAH, pulmonary arterial hypertension.

Adapted from Simonneau G, Robbins IM, Beghetti M, et al. Updated clinical classification of pulmonary hypertension. J Am Coll Cardiol 2009;54(Suppl 1):S43–54; with permission.

precapillary pulmonary vessels, thus increasing the pulmonary vascular resistance.[20] It has been observed that there are elevated levels of ET-1 in patients with PH and these elevations correlate with the PH severity.[20] Vasoconstriction from alveolar hypoxia and resulting endothelial dysfunction seems to be the major stimulus for overexpression of ET-1.[19]

Endothelial dysfunction also causes impaired production of NO.[19] NO is a potent vasodilator, smooth muscle cell regulator, and platelet inhibitor.[21] In pulmonary vasculature, it is synthesized by endothelial nitric oxide synthetase (eNOS), whose activity is effected by stimuli, such as hypoxia, inflammation, and oxidative stress.[21] Downregulation of the eNOS-NO-cyclic guanosine monophosphate (cGMP) pathway results in pulmonary vasoconstriction and increase in pulmonary vascular resistance.[21] Endogenous NO production is also affected by the binding of ET-1 to ETB receptors and is the rationale for investigations of selective ETA receptor inhibition in the treatment of PH.[21]

There is involvement of additional inflammatory pathways affecting the pulmonary vasculature in both IPAH and CTD-related APAH; these are more pronounced in the latter, perhaps contributing to the observed differences in treatment response and survival.[2] The activation of platelets, disturbances in the coagulation cascade, and abnormal thrombolysis have also been observed to contribute to the development and progression of PAH.[18] Disordered proteolysis of the extracellular matrix is also evident in PAH.[18] Histologically, the lesions in both IPAH and CTD-related PAH appear quite similar.[2,17] There is medial hypertrophy due to hypoxemia and vasoconstriction, intimal proliferation, and, later on, obliteration of vessels.[2,22] Plexiform lesions, which are glomeruloid complex vascular structures originating from pulmonary arteries, may be present in severe PAH. Plexiform lesions are made up of a core of mesenchymal cells, smooth muscle cells, and apoptosis-resistant myofibroblasts surrounded by a proliferating network of vascular channels.[23] Certain hormones, like estrogen, have been considered as having a potential role in the pathogenesis of PAH by promoting cellular proliferation and smooth muscle proliferation.[5] This may, at least in part, account for the gender differences seen in the prevalence and natural history of some forms of PH.[24] In CTD, the pulmonary parenchymal disease may lead to isolated medial hypertrophy in the precapillary pulmonary arterial bed with or without concurrent intimal fibrosis.[17]

CLINICAL PRESENTATION

The most frequent initial symptom, seen in up to 60% of the PAH patient population, is dyspnea on exertion.[5,17,18,25] This may be a result of hypoxia, cardiac dysfunction, and/or limitation to the cardiac output, which can be generated during exertion.[17] By the time of diagnosis, more than 90% of patients will be noting dyspnea on exertion (or will be limiting their exertion to avoid the sensation of dyspnea). Approximately 50% of patients will ultimately complain of exertional chest discomfort, which can be due to right ventricular ischemia occurring because the right ventricle has increased muscle mass and is under strain.[17,18,25,26] Other symptoms that occur in severe PH and ultimately in right heart failure are seen later in the course of disease and may include exertional presyncope, syncope, abdominal distension, peripheral edema, right upper quadrant abdominal pain, early satiety, hemoptysis, and hoarseness (due to compression of the left recurrent laryngeal nerve between the aorta and the left pulmonary artery [Ortner syndrome]).[17,18,25,26] A delay in PAH diagnosis (several PAH registries have found a mean of 2+ years from onset of symptoms to establishment of a diagnosis) and therefore in treatment is mainly because the initial symptoms may occur only with exertion, and are nonspecific, and more specific or obvious symptoms may not manifest until late in the disease process.[5,26,27] This may be because the normal pulmonary circulation has significant reserve (for recruitment and distention) and can accommodate large changes in flow with little or no change in pressures.[17]

On examination of the patient, early findings may include a dominant a-wave in the jugular venous pulse; with disease progression, this a-wave becomes less prominent and the v-wave becomes larger.[17] Cardiac examination is often remarkable for a loud P2 and a narrow split of S2. With advancement of disease, a right-sided S3 or S4 may become audible. A murmur of tricuspid regurgitation may often be heard on left sternal border; this murmur is higher pitched than the tricuspid regurgitation murmur noted in intrinsic tricuspid valvular disease. Other remarkable findings may include persistent hypoxia not responsive to oxygen supplementation and peripheral cyanosis.[17]

DIAGNOSIS

PH carries with it significant morbidity and a high mortality; therefore, the goal is to have early detection and treatment of the disease.[28] The suspicion and confirmation of the diagnosis of PH can involve several different testing modalities.[29] Testing can be divided into screening for PH, confirming the diagnosis and type of PH (ie, PAH), evaluating for disease severity, and assessing for etiology.[30]

Screening

Transthoracic echocardiography (TTE) is an essential tool and the noninvasive investigation of choice for screening for suspected PH.[31,32] Echocardiography can be used to estimate PA systolic pressures, to evaluate right ventricle size and function, to evaluate the left side of the heart, to assess tricuspid annular plane systolic excursion (TAPSE, a measure of right ventricular contractility), to assess valve function and to determine the presence of valvular stenosis or regurgitation, to measure size and function of all the cardiac chambers, and to determine the presence and size of a pericardial effusion.[26,28,33] Agitated saline as contrast injection can be used to improve detection of right to left shunting while performing a TTE.[26] TTE can also serve as a tool for patient follow-up and monitoring responses to therapy.[18,31,32] TTE has been found to have a higher sensitivity (82%) and specificity (69%) for the diagnosis of PH when compared with magnetic resonance imaging (MRI) and pulmonary function tests (PFTs).[28] The data on the combination of other noninvasive modalities with TTE to increase the accuracy of detection on PH is scarce and needs further study.[28]

Confirmation

Right heart catheterization (RHC) is the gold standard for the diagnosis of PH and to distinguish PAH from other forms of PH. It can allow accurate determination of the pulmonary arterial pressures, the pulmonary capillary wedge pressure (PCWP), and the cardiac output and is necessary for the calculation of pulmonary vascular resistance (PVR).[28] It allows determination of hemodynamic parameters with precision, thus playing an important role in prognostication.[18] With measurement of the PCWP (as a surrogate for left atrial pressure) it can establish the contribution of the left side of the heart to the etiology of PH. With other measurements (ie, right atrial pressure [RAP] and cardiac output [CO]), it allows determination of the severity of the PH, and its effect on right heart function. RHC also allows for a vasodilator trial that assesses the capacity of the pulmonary vessels to vasodilate.[18] Inhaled NO, prostacyclins (intravenous [IV] and inhaled) and IV adenosine have been used in vasodilator trials to evaluate for pulmonary arterial vasoreactivity.[26] A favorable vasodilator response is presently defined as a reduction in mPAP by at least 10 mm Hg, to a value less than or equal to 40 mm Hg, with a maintained or increased cardiac output.[34] Very few patients with CTD-PAH are found to be significantly vasoreactive.

Severity and Prognosis

TTE can be used not only for screening for PH, but also for assessing for its severity and prognosis. The measurement of parameters such as right atrial area, right ventricular size function, TAPSE, and pericardial effusion can be used to determine the severity of the PH.[33,35] A TAPSE smaller than 1.7 cm signifies worse right ventricular (RV) function and has been associated with a higher mortality.[33] Similarly, presence of a moderate (10–20 mm) to large (>20 mm) size pericardial effusion signifies right heart failure with an elevated right atrial pressure, and has been associated with a higher mortality.[35,36]

Chest radiograph may reveal enlargement of either the pulmonary arteries or the RV, but these are usually observed later in the disease course.[17,26] Electrocardiogram will show an RV strain pattern and right axis deviation in advanced disease when RV hypertrophy has occurred.[26]

Exercise capacity testing by 6-minute walk test will provide an inexpensive and reproducible assessment of a patient's physical capacity and determine the time and distance at which oxygen desaturation occurs (and its severity).[26] It can serve as the objective basis for a home oxygen prescription. Although the 6-minute walk test has proven reliable in assessing patients with IPAH, its reliability in scleroderma remains controversial.[37,38]

A cardiopulmonary exercise test will reveal impaired gas exchange and decreased exercise tolerance with an abnormal increase in dead space ventilation in PH.[26] The pattern of abnormalities will resemble a cardiac limitation to exercise rather than a respiratory limitation.[39]

Laboratory testing can reveal abnormal hepatic enzymes signifying liver congestion, or polycythemia, a consequence of chronic hypoxia and elevation of atrial natriuretic peptide and uric acid signifying heart failure.[29] According to a study by Heresi and colleagues,[40] elevated plasma cardiac troponin I (cTnI), even at subclinically detectable levels, is associated with more severe disease and worse outcomes in patients with PAH. Other bio markers that have significant prognostic value include circulating red cell distribution width (RDW), growth differentiation factor 15, interleukin-6, creatinine, brain natriutetic peptide (BNP) and NT-proBNP levels; studies have shown that these may be used to predict survival in patients with IPAH.[41,42]

Etiology

Noninvasive investigations used in diagnosing and determining the etiology of a patient with PH include PFTs, high-resolution computerized tomography (HRCT), CT angiography, ventilation perfusion scan (VQ Scan), chest MRI, cardiovascular magnetic resonance (CMR), and pulmonary scintigraphy.[18,29,30,43]

Invasive procedures that can be used in the diagnosis of PH include pulmonary artery arteriography, which remains the most definitive test for the diagnosis and mapping of chronic, unresolved pulmonary emboli.[44] Lung biopsy has little to add as a diagnostic and prognostic modality in patients with PH and its use is limited because of the morbidity and mortality associated with the procedure in these patients.[45]

Laboratory tests that are important in diagnosis of CTD-related PH include antinuclear antibody, anticardiolipin antibody, erythrocyte sedimentation rate, rheumatoid factor, anti-Scleroderma 70 antibody (Anti Scl 70 Ab), and Sjogren antibody (SS-A, SS-B).[26]

DIAGNOSTIC WORKUP IN CTD APAH

The investigations done in CTD APAH are similar to the modalities generally used in evaluating other etiologies of PH but there are some variations to be noted.

Criteria to use echocardiography in screening for PH in relatively asymptomatic patients are different for various CTDs and are related to the disease prevalence of PH observed in these disorders.[46,47]

In a study by Rajaram and colleagues,[48] tricuspid regurgitant gradient as measured by TTE and ventricular mass index as measured by MRI had greater correlation with mPAP and PVR as measured by RHC in CTD APAH patients whereas CT appears to be limited as a diagnostic and prognostic tool for PH in these patients.

PH IN CTD

The pathogenesis of PH in connective tissue disease appears to be similar to that of IPAH.[49] Endothelial dysfunction leads to myofibroblast activation and subsequent vasoconstriction and smooth muscle hypertrophy.[50] There is increased production of endothelin and decreased production of nitric oxide and prostacyclins, which causes inflammation and fibrosis of small and medium-sized pulmonary arteries leading to increased resistance in pulmonary vasculature.[50] The incidence of APAH in different connective tissue disorders and the known associations or risk factors for developing CTD APAH are presented in **Table 2**.

Badesch and colleagues[5] and Chung and colleagues[51] have analyzed the data from the recent REVEAL Registry, which was established to characterize the clinical course, treatment, and predictors of outcomes in patients with PAH in the United States. This registry is the largest US cohort of patients with PAH confirmed by right-sided heart catheterization (RHC), and contains a substantial number of patients with CTD-PAH.[5,51] Of the enrolled patients with PAH in this registry from 54 US centers, 50.7% of the patients had APAH, whereas 46.2% had IPAH.[5] Among the associated patients with PH, 49.9% was CTD related, which highlights the clinical occurrence of this particular entity.[5] In APAH in this registry of patients, there was an observed female-to-male prevalence of 3.8:1.0.[5] Chung and colleagues[51] analyzed

Table 2
Prevalence of pulmonary hypertension/pulmonary arterial hypertension and risk factors in connective tissue disease

Connective Tissue Disease	Prevalence	Risk Factors
Scleroderma	7%–27%	Low DLCO
Systemic lupus erythematosus	0.5%–43%	LAC, pregnancy
Sjogren syndrome	Rare	Anti-Ro/SSA Ab, Anti-RNP Ab, RF, hypergammaglobulinemia
Rheumatoid arthritis	Rare	—
Mixed connective tissue disease	50%–60%	—
Polymyositis/dermatomyositis	25%	—

Abbreviations: Ab, antibody; DLCO, carbon monoxide diffusion capacity; LAC, lupus anticoagulant; RF, rheumatoid factor; RNP, ribonucleoprotein; Ro, part of ribonucleoprotein; SSA, Sjogren syndrome A.

1-year mortality from the time of registry enrollment in patients with CTD APAH and compared those with systemic sclerosis (SSc) with those with systemic lupus erythematosus (SLE), mixed connective tissue disease (MCTD), and rheumatoid arthritis (RA). SSc-related APAH had the worst 1-year survival at 82% versus 94% in SLE APAH, 88% in MCTD APAH, and 96% in RA APAH.[51]

SCLERODERMA

The lung is currently the fourth most commonly involved organ in scleroderma, after skin, peripheral arterial vessels, and the esophagus.[31] The pulmonary involvement is most frequently in the form of either interstitial lung disease or pulmonary vascular disease.[31] The prevalence of PH in SSc is estimated to be 7% to 27%.[52] In the United States, of all patients with SSc, about 10% suffer from PAH, making it more common than any other form of PAH in the World Health Organization group 1, including IPAH.[52] There is concern that many patients with scleroderma-associated PAH are not suspected of having the condition, and that it is underdiagnosed and undertreated. The 1-year survival rate of patients with SSc-related PAH had been approximately 45% (before the current era of PAH therapies), as compared with the survival of patients with SSc who have parenchymal lung involvement (ie, interstitial lung disease) without PAH who had a 1-year survival rate of approximately 90%.[50,53,54] With newer PAH therapies, the 1-year survival rate for patients with SSc APAH has increased to about 80% (emphasizing the importance of both appropriate diagnosis, and early treatment).[53,55]

The patients with scleroderma with lower carbon monoxide diffusion capacity (DLCO) and higher BNP are more at risk of clinically manifesting PAH.[46,52] The symptoms of PAH are unfortunately nonspecific and are similar to those observed in ILD, most commonly exertional dyspnea and fatigue.[50,52] The symptoms of PAH in patients with SSc also can be confused with similar symptoms caused by the anemia, or muscle and skin involvement that occurs in scleroderma. Concomitant renal and myocardial dysfunctions are important predictors of mortality in SSc.[55] Patients with scleroderma can have depressed RV function as well as left ventricle systolic and/ or diastolic dysfunction.[56] SSc-APAH patients also have a higher prevalence of pericardial effusion (up to 34%), as compared with IPAH patients (at about 13%).[55] In PAH, the presence of a pericardial effusion is felt to be associated with right ventricular failure, and predicts a poorer prognosis.[55] Literature has suggested annual screening of all patients with scleroderma with transthoracic echocardiograms for detecting PH, as it has such high prevalence and morbidity.[47]

In scleroderma, interstitial changes in pulmonary parenchyma can be detected with HRCT at early stages of the disease when chest radiographs may be still appear to be normal.[31]

According to Hesselstrand and colleagues,[43] CMR in patients with APAH with scleroderma often demonstrates severe pathology with decrease in the RV end diastolic volume (RVEDV) and reduction in ejection fraction (RVEF), as well as fibrosis at the insertion point of right ventricle as compared with patients with scleroderma but not PAH who show less severe changes. Further studies are needed to see if these findings can be of value in screening for early signs of PAH in patients with SSc.[43]

The sensitivity of PFTs for diagnosis of PAH in scleroderma is approximately 70%, as reported by Hsu and colleagues.[15] PFTs may show decrease in DLCO and forced vital capacity (FVC) of similar magnitude in patients with interstitial lung disease. The DLCO may decrease at a more rapid rate than FVC in pulmonary vascular disease (PH) occurring without concurrent interstitial lung disease; this results in a high FVC (percent predicted)/DLCO (percent predicted) ratio.[31] Patients with scleroderma with FVC/DLCO ratios greater than 1 are more likely to have PAH as compared with ratios of 1 or lower who are more likely to have interstitial lung disease.[31,57]

SLE

SLE involves various organs of the body, including skin, joints, kidney, blood, heart, and lungs. Pulmonary involvement in SLE can be in the form of pleuritis, parenchymal involvement (such as lymphoid interstitial pneumonia), bronchiolitis obliterans with organizing pneumonia, vascular involvement including PH, acute reversible hypoxemia, alveolar hemorrhage, antiphospholipid syndrome, or muscular and diaphragmatic involvement causing shrinking lung syndrome.[53,58] The reported prevalence of PAH in SLE ranges from 0.5% to 43.0%.[46] The wide variation is seen as most of the studies have been on small cohorts with different definitions of PAH and use of different diagnostic methods.[46] The presence of lupus anticoagulant (LAC) is a major risk factor for developing venous thromboembolism and PAH in patients with SLE.[46] In SLE, the risk of developing PAH does not correlate with DLCO, as it does in SSc.[46,53] If PAH develops in SLE, it is often associated with rapid deterioration and poor prognosis.[46] The role of screening for PAH in SLE is still under question but literature suggests screening in asymptomatic patients with risk factors such as a positive LAC or if they are planning pregnancy.[46] PAH in SLE appears to more frequently respond to treatment with immunosuppressants and corticosteroids than do other forms of PAH.[59]

SJOGREN SYNDROME

Sjogren syndrome (SS) is a chronic inflammatory disease largely affecting lacrimal and salivary glands. The pulmonary complications in SS are mainly manifested as small airways and interstitial lung disease.[60] The occurrence of PAH in SS is rare and only a few patients have been reported in the literature to date. The patient population in one study was exclusively female and had a mean age at diagnosis of 50 years.[2,60] The prevalence of PAH in SS seems to be associated with increased frequency of the presence of anti-Ro/SSA antibodies, anti-ribonucleoprotein (RNP) antibodies, rheumatoid factor, and hypergammaglobulinemia, suggesting that autoimmune mechanisms may be playing a role in PH pathogenesis.[60]

RHEUMATOID ARTHRITIS

Rheumatoid arthritis (RA) is usually associated with synovial inflammation but can also involve extra-articular organs of the body, such as skin, lungs, blood vessels, and the central and peripheral nervous system. PAH is a rare complication of RA.[2] The pulmonary artery (PA) pressures are most commonly elevated in RA secondary to interstitial fibrosis and pulmonary vasculitis, with resultant medial and intimal thickening.[17] Infrequently, pulmonary vasculitis may occur in the absence of parenchymal lung involvement, in these cases prognosis is grave.[17]

MCTD

MCTD is a condition that manifests overlapping features of SLE, RA, and scleroderma with presence of anti-RNP antibodies.[17,56] In some cases, the pathologic findings consist of necrotizing vasculitis, whereas in others intimal fibrosis, fibrin thrombi, and plexiform vasculopathy may be seen.[17] The prevalence of PAH has been reported to be as high as 50% to 60% in this disorder.[17,56] Data on prognosis with current management options are limited.

POLYMYOSITIS/DERMATOMYOSITIS

Polymyositis/dermatomyositis is characterized by inflammation of the skeletal muscles causing muscular weakness and elevation of creatinine kinase and aldolase.[61] It can be associated with skin involvement to cause Gottron papules (scaly erythematous eruptions or red patches overlying the knuckles, elbows, and knees) and the heliotrope rash (purple rash over the upper eyelids) characteristic of dermatomyositis. Lung involvement occurs in the form of aspiration pneumonia, acute or chronic respiratory failure, hypoventilation due to diaphragmatic myopathy, diffuse interstitial pneumonia, acute interstitial pneumonia, and occasionally as PH.[17,61,62] The development of interstitial pneumonitis occurs in about 30% to 47% of the cases and carries a grave prognosis.[17,61,62] One autopsy series found evidence of plexiform vasculopathy in as many as 25% of the patients suffering from polymyositis regardless of whether or not they had clinical manifestations of PAH.[17]

TREATMENT

PAH in CTD is a challenging disease and complex to manage medically.[17,63,64] The treatment guidelines are modeled on the principles of treating IPAH group 1 PAH.[65] These conditions had a poor prognosis through the mid-1980s when the modalities of treatment were limited to supportive measures and occasionally (in responders only) calcium channel blockers.[17,63,66] As new therapies have been developed targeting specific pathways of PAH pathogenesis, the survival rates have improved.[17,63,66] These novel therapies have also played an important role in improving patients' symptoms and quality of life as well as their mortality.[63,66]

In addition to specific modalities of treatment, the disease is managed by eliminating any possible causative factors.[17] Important supportive measures include oxygen supplementation, use of low-salt diet, diuretics, inotropic agents, calcium channel blockers in vasoreactive disease, and anticoagulation.[17,63,66–68]

With advancement in the PAH treatment options, there are presently 3 major classes of medications that are available in the United States for use as monotherapy and/or combination therapy.[66,68,69] These target the prostacyclin, endothelin, and NO-mediated pathways involved in the pathophysiology of the disease process.[68–70] A summary of current treatment modalities is given in **Fig. 1**.

PROSTACYCLIN ANALOGUES

Prostacyclin production requires an enzyme prostacyclin synthase, which is deficient in patients with PAH.[70] The deficiency of prostacyclin has been linked with the vascular changes observed in PAH, namely thrombosis, vasoconstriction, and proliferation of vascular smooth muscle.[70–73] Using synthetic prostacyclin and its analogues as a treatment for PAH can result in the reversal of these changes, as these agents have strong vasodilator and antiproliferative properties, mediating them by increasing cyclic AMP via activation of adenylate cyclase.[64,65,70–74]

The agents that have been studied in clinical trials include epoprostenol, treprostinil, iloprost, beraprost, and selexipag.[65,66,70–72,74,75] Beraprost is an oral prostacyclin analogue, and selexipag is an oral (nonprostanoid) selective prostacyclin receptor (IP receptor) agonist, neither has yet been approved for use in the United States.

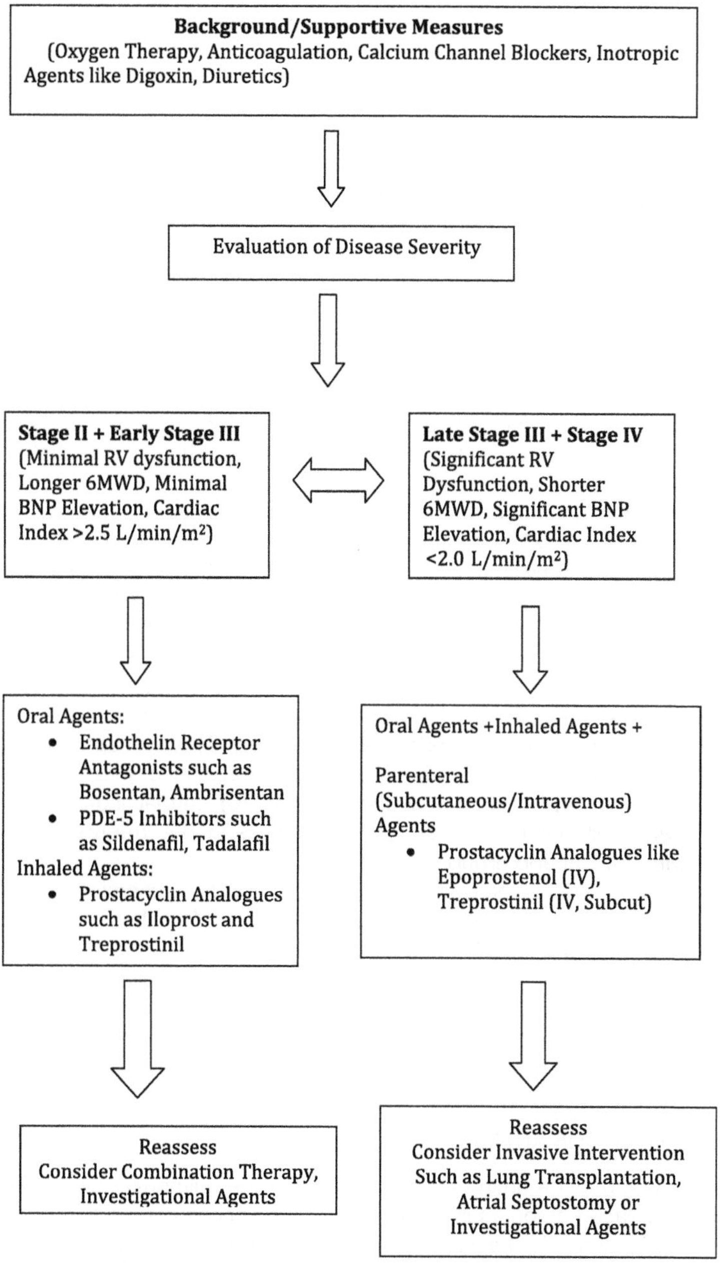

Background/Supportive Measures
(Oxygen Therapy, Anticoagulation, Calcium Channel Blockers, Inotropic Agents like Digoxin, Diuretics)

Evaluation of Disease Severity

Stage II + Early Stage III
(Minimal RV dysfunction, Longer 6MWD, Minimal BNP Elevation, Cardiac Index >2.5 L/min/m²)

Late Stage III + Stage IV
(Significant RV Dysfunction, Shorter 6MWD, Significant BNP Elevation, Cardiac Index <2.0 L/min/m²)

Oral Agents:
- Endothelin Receptor Antagonists such as Bosentan, Ambrisentan
- PDE-5 Inhibitors such as Sildenafil, Tadalafil

Inhaled Agents:
- Prostacyclin Analogues such as Iloprost and Treprostinil

Oral Agents +Inhaled Agents +

Parenteral (Subcutaneous/Intravenous) Agents
- Prostacyclin Analogues like Epoprostenol (IV), Treprostinil (IV, Subcut)

Reassess
Consider Combination Therapy, Investigational Agents

Reassess
Consider Invasive Intervention Such as Lung Transplantation, Atrial Septostomy or Investigational Agents

Fig. 1. Treatment algorithm. (*Adapted from* McLaughlin VV, Archer SL, Badesch DB, et al. ACCF/AHA 2009 expert consensus document on pulmonary hypertension a report of the American College of Cardiology Foundation Task Force on expert consensus documents and the American Heart Association developed in collaboration with the American College of Chest Physicians; American Thoracic Society, Inc.; and the Pulmonary Hypertension Association. J Am Coll Cardiol 2009;53(17):1573–619; with permission.)

In 1995, epoprostenol was the first agent to be approved for treatment of PAH (IPAH) in the United States.[71] It was subsequently (in 1999) specifically approved for use in PAH associated with scleroderma by the US Food and Drug Administration (FDA).[64] This drug has a very short half life and requires constant IV infusion; therefore, it is reserved for patients with more advanced symptoms and disease.[63,76] Studies by Barst and colleagues,[77,78] McLaughlin and colleagues,[79-81] Humbert and colleagues,[82,83] Badesch and colleagues, and Simonneau and colleagues have shown improvement in factors such as exercise tolerance, cardiac output, and vascular resistance, as well as improvement in survival rates at short-term and long-term time points in patients being treated with this agent. A study by Badesch and colleagues[84] on 102 patients with scleroderma-associated PAH (functional class III and IV) showed improved survival as compared with the natural history of the disease. Initially, IV epoprostenol was thought of as a bridge to lung transplantation in patients with severe PH (New York Heart Association functional class III and IV) but now is considered a chronic therapeutic agent for long-term administration for functional class IV patients and is also used in functional class IV patients who are not suitable candidates for lung transplantation.[85,86]

Treprostinil is a longer acting, more stable prostacyclin analogue that was approved in the United States in 2002 for continuous subcutaneous treatment of functional class II, III, and IV PAH.[63,71] It was subsequently approved for use as a continuous IV infusion therapy in 2004. It has potent antithrombotic and vasodilator properties and because of a longer half-life than epoprostenol, can also be administered by inhalational routes.[63,71] It was approved in the United States as an inhalational agent to improve exercise capacity in patients with PAH in functional class III in 2009.[65] Oudiz and colleagues[64] studied 90 patients with CTD and PAH, including patients with SLE, diffuse scleroderma, limited scleroderma, and mixed CTD/overlap syndrome who were treated with either continuous subcutaneous treprostinil or placebo. The results showed improvement in 6-minute walk distance (6MWD), cardiac index, dyspnea and fatigue scores, and pulmonary vascular resistance in the treprostinil group as compared with the placebo group.[64]

Iloprost was approved in the United States in 2004 and is a chemically stable prostacyclin analogue that can be administered as an aerosol.[65,71] It is more selective to the pulmonary circulation due to its mode of administration, but the frequency of dosing (needs to be taken 6 to 9 times a day) may cause compliance issues.[66,71]

Common adverse effects of all prostacyclin analogues include headache, flushing, nausea, jaw pain, infusion site pain with subcutaneous administration, and risk of catheter infection with IV administration.[71]

ENDOTHELIN-RECEPTOR ANTAGONISTS

Endothelin-1 is a peptide amino acid expressed in the pulmonary circulation that is secreted in increased amounts in PAH.[63,73,87,88] Its actions are mediated by 2 types of receptors: ET_A and ET_B. It acts on vascular endothelium to cause vasoconstriction as well as on vascular smooth muscle to cause proliferation.[73,86,88] To target these actions, oral endothelin receptor antagonists have been developed. Bosentan is a nonselective endothelin receptor antagonist, whereas ambrisentan may be relatively selective to ET_A at lower doses. In a randomized, double-blind, placebo-controlled trial of bosentan by Channick and colleagues[89] (consisting of 32 patients with PAH of which 5 patients had scleroderma-related PAH), bosentan resulted in significant improvement in hemodynamics and 6MWD as compared to placebo. In a subsequent study by Rubin and colleagues[90] of 213 patients with PAH in functional classes III and

IV (including 80 patients with scleroderma-related PAH and 25 patients with SLE-related PAH), bosentan showed improvement in exercise capacity, functional class, and time to clinical worsening and the effect was more pronounced with the higher-studied dose. Currently, bosentan is approved in the United States for use in functional class II, III, and IV PAH.[63,89–91] Side effects of bosentan include headache, flushing, dizziness and syncope, and elevated liver transaminases.[51]

Ambrisentan has shown improvement in 6MWD after 12 weeks of treatment in published clinical trials.[92] The studies included 41 and 40 patients with CTD-related PAH in ARIES 1 (202 patients) and ARIES-2 (192 patients), respectively.[92] Peripheral edema and congestive heart failure have been reported with its use.[92]

Macitentan is a new oral ET (A & B) receptor antagonist that has recently completed a large event-driven phase III clinical trial.[93] It is currently undergoing FDA review.

PHOSPHODIESTERASE 5 INHIBITORS

NO acts via cyclic GMP to cause vasodilation and to inhibit cellular proliferation, and its impaired production in patients with PH is one factor contributing to the vasoconstriction and cellular proliferation of the diseased pulmonary vascular bed.[63,70,76] Phosphodiestrase-5 (PDE-5) inhibitors work by inhibiting the action of the PDE-5 enzyme on degradation of cyclic GMP; this effectively increases the activity of NO, thus facilitating pulmonary vascular dilatation.[56,70] Sildenafil has been most widely studied in this class of drugs and has shown improvement in PAH hemodynamics and clinical symptoms with oral use.[94–96] It was approved in 2005 for use in IPAH functional class II and III patients (at a dosage of 20 mg 3 times a day).[65] Trials by Zhao and colleagues,[97] Sastry and colleagues,[98] and Wilkins and colleagues[99] looked at its efficacy and found that in a dose-dependent manner, it decreased mPAP, and increased exercise capacity and 6MWD.[96] In 2007, an analysis of patients with CTD-related PAH from the SUPER-1 study of oral sildenafil for 12 weeks, confirmed the improvement in hemodynamics, functional capacity, and exercise capacity in patients with CTD-related PAH.[100] Currently, sildenafil is considered by some to be the drug of choice in patients with scleroderma with PAH because of ease of administration and low incidence of side effects.[56]

Tadalafil is another PDE-5 inhibitor that was approved for use in PAH in 2009 by the FDA.[101,102] It is dosed once daily and has side effects such as headache, flushing, diarrhea, and nasal congestion.[101,102] Its use has shown sustained improvements in 6MWD.[103]

INVESTIGATIONAL AGENTS
Tyrosine Kinase Inhibitors

Tyrosine kinase inhibitors have been used as antineoplastic drugs in chronic myelogenous leukemia, renal cell carcinoma, colon cancer, and hepatocellular carcinoma but now their use is being studied for nonmalignant processes, such as diabetes, glomerulonephritis, cardiac hypertrophy, rheumatoid disorders, and PH.[104] The proliferation of pulmonary vasculature in PAH is similar to neoplastic vascular proliferation, although lacking the properties of metastasis and invasion.[105] There is increased expression of PDGF and VEGF in PAH, which is the therapeutic target in this class of drugs.[56,105] In a double-blind, randomized, placebo-controlled trial by Ghofrani and colleagues,[106] imatinib was given to 59 patients with class II to IV PAH. Patients with more severe disease showed improvement in pulmonary vascular resistance and cardiac output but there was no change in 6MWD. This was a phase II trial and more studies are needed to establish efficacy and safety of the different tyrosine kinase inhibitors in this patient population. There has been a concern for subdural hematomas in patients receiving imatinib.[107,108]

Guanylate Cyclase Stimulators

Riociguat is an investigational agent that stimulates soluble guanylate cyclase (sGC) and synergizes with endogenous NO to activate the NO-sGC-cGMP pathway and cause increased production of cGMP.[109–111] The cGMP in turn causes vasodilation of the pulmonary vasculature.[110] The Phase III, double-blind, randomized, placebo-controlled PATENT-1 study to investigate the efficacy and safety of riociguat in patients with symptomatic PAH has been completed and has shown good efficacy, favorable pharmacokinetics, and tolerability.[109–112] The FDA has recently approved the application of riociguat (Adampas) for the treatment of Group 1 PAH and Group 4 chronic thromboembolic pulmonary hypertension (CTEPH).

NO

NO is administered as a continuous gas (nasal) inhalation. It is active in the pulmonary circulation and activates guanylate cyclase and converts it into cGMP, which in turn acts as a vasodilator of pulmonary circulation.[113] NO is useful as a selective vasodilator of pulmonary circulation, as it is directly delivered in the pulmonary circulation via inhalation.[113] It has been approved by the FDA only for treatment of acute hypoxic respiratory failure in term neonates but has been used off-label as a therapeutic agent in PH.[113] Additional studies of NO and related compounds are ongoing.

COMBINATION OF DRUG GROUPS

There are very few data to date regarding the use of combination therapy in either IPAH, APAH, or CTD-APAH. Guidelines suggest combination therapy for patients who fail or symptomatically progress on monotherapy.[114] Combination therapy is beneficial, as the drugs may act synergistically by targeting multiple disease pathways.[69] In an observational study by Kemp and colleagues,[115] 16 functional class III and 7 class IV patients were analyzed for efficacy and safety of upfront combination epoprostenol and bosentan therapy. The upfront combination therapy with epoprostenol and bosentan was found to be associated with improvements in important outcomes, such as functional class, exercise capacity, and hemodynamics.[115] The PACES (Pulmonary Arterial Hypertension Combination Study of Epoprostenol and Sildenafil) trial in 2008 concluded that addition of sildenafil to chronic IV epoprostenol therapy improved exercise capacity, hemodynamic parameters, time to clinical worsening, and quality of life.[116] A recent meta-analysis by Fox and colleagues[117] found that when compared with monotherapy, combination therapy improved exercise capacity modestly but does not offer any benefit otherwise. The BREATHE-2 trial, which was a placebo-controlled, double-blind prospective study published in 2004, showed a trend toward improved hemodynamics upon combining bosentan with epoprostenol in patients with severe PH who were either idiopathic or CTD related.[118] This study did not reach statistical significance because of the small number of patients involved. Interestingly, there was a low incidence of side effects, such as jaw pain and hypotension when epoprostenol was used in combination with bosentan.[118] The TRIUMPH-1 trial by McLaughlin and colleagues[119] demonstrated that addition of inhaled treprostinil to oral bosentan or sildenafil in patients who remain symptomatic on these initial drugs improved quality of life and exercise capacity (6MWD) with statistical significance, and was well tolerated. Patients included in this study carried a diagnosis of either idiopathic, familial, CTD-associated, HIV-associated, or anorexigen-associated PAH.

LUNG TRANSPLANTATION

Lung transplantation is the last resort treatment for severe PH refractory to treatment with oral, inhaled, and particularly subcutaneous and IV drugs.[120] Due to the current availability of multiple drugs for the treatment of PAH, the proportion of patients undergoing lung transplantation for PAH has decreased to one-third of what it was previously.[121] Patients are now usually referred for lung transplantation with Class IV heart failure and median life expectancy of less than 2 years.[120,121] Criteria for referring for a transplant are worsening hemodynamics, including mPAP higher than 55 mm Hg, systolic systemic arterial pressure lower than120 mm Hg, cardiac index less than 2 L/min/m^2, central venous pressure higher than 15 mm Hg or functional parameters (peak oxygen uptake <10–12 mL/kg/min, 6MWD <332 m) as they correlate with mortality.[122] Patients with PAH most commonly undergo bilateral lung transplantation, whereas some patients with severe right ventricular failure may require heart lung transplantation.[120,121] Current studies provide data favoring bilateral lung transplantation as the procedure of choice for patients with PAH when comparing the functional recovery, hospital/intensive care unit stay, pulmonary pressures, and incidence of acute/chronic rejection with the results following single lung transplantation and heart-lung transplantations.[121] Patients with connective tissue disease may not be optimal candidates for lung transplantation because of multiorgan involvement and morbidity specifically due to esophageal dysmotility and renal involvement; they need proper screening to assess for their potentially increased risk of posttransplantation complications.[66] It is of note that studies have shown decreased survival in patients with scleroderma after lung transplantation as compared with a patient population with other systemic diseases undergoing the same transplantation, so epoprostenol remains a valuable alternative long-term therapy for these patients.[123–125]

SUMMARY

PAH associated with connective tissue diseases is associated with significant functional impairment and morbidity, and carries with it a poor prognosis.[126,127] The mortality is as high as 10% to 15% in the first year after diagnosis; making it a devastating disease.[1] The availability of ever-increasing numbers of treatment options in the recent era have improved survival in this patient population and have made early and accurate diagnosis a more important goal.[126,127] According to the Registry to Evaluate Early and Long-Term Pulmonary Arterial Hypertension Disease Management (REVEAL), 1-year, 3-year, 5-year, and 7-year survival rates from time of diagnostic right-sided heart catheterization in patients with PAH were found to be 85%, 68%, 57%, and 49%, respectively, which is a considerable improvement since the National Institutes of Health registry 2 decades previously.[128] In a study by Condliffe and colleagues,[127] survival rates in patients with SSC-associated PAH have improved to 78% at 1 year and 47% at 3 years. Patients with SLE-related PAH have a much higher survival rate of up to 75% at 3 years. Proper screening, early diagnosis, and early treatment can have a significant impact in reducing morbidity and mortality. A small study to assess outcomes in patients with asymptomatic CTD found to have exercise induced PAH suggest that bosentan may be safe and effective in improving the hemodynamics and outcomes in these patients.[129] This study included only 10 patients, and additional randomized trials with larger numbers of subjects are needed to affirm this hypothesis. Studies are under way to find additional therapeutic modalities in the form of PDGF receptor blockers, VEGF blockers, tyrosine kinase inhibitors, endothelial dysfunction inhibitors, multikinase inhibitor of Raf-1, serotonin receptor antagonists, and rho kinase inhibitors.[130,131] Despite these, clinical suspicion, early diagnosis, early treatment, and referral to specialized centers of expertise remain the best hope for patients at the present time.

REFERENCES

1. Vogel-Claussen J, Skrok J, Shehata ML, et al. Right and left ventricular myocardial perfusion reserves correlate with right ventricular function and pulmonary hemodynamics in patients with pulmonary arterial hypertension. Radiology 2011;258(1):119–27.
2. Hassoun PM. Pulmonary arterial hypertension complicating connective tissue diseases. Semin Respir Crit Care Med 2009;30(4):429–39.
3. Opitz CF, Blindt R, Blumberg F, et al. Pulmonary hypertension: hemodynamic evaluation: hemodynamic evaluation—recommendations of the Cologne Consensus Conference 2010. Dtsch Med Wochenschr 2010;135(Suppl 3):S78–86.
4. Montani D, Chaouat A. Diagnosis and classification of pulmonary hypertension. Presse Med 2010;39(Suppl 1):1S3–15.
5. Badesch DB, Raskob GE, Elliott CG, et al. Pulmonary arterial hypertension: baseline characteristics from the REVEAL Registry. Chest 2010;137(2):376–87.
6. Hoeper MM. Definition, classification, and epidemiology of pulmonary arterial hypertension. Semin Respir Crit Care Med 2009;30(4):369–75.
7. Kovacs G, Olschewski H. Pulmonary arterial pressure during rest and exercise (from Geneva, 1961 to Dana Point, 2008). Annals of Respiratory Medicine 2010; 1(2).
8. Simonneau G. A new clinical classification of pulmonary hypertension. Bull Acad Natl Med 2009;193(8):1897–909.
9. Rich S. Primary pulmonary hypertension: executive summary from the World Symposium (Evian, France - 1998). 1998. Available at: http://www.who.int/ncd/cvd/pph.htm. Accessed August 1, 2013.
10. Fishman AP. Clinical classification of pulmonary hypertension. Clin Chest Med 2001;22(3):385–91, vii.
11. Humbert M, Nunes H, Sitbon O, et al. Risk factors for pulmonary arterial hypertension. Clin Chest Med 2001;22(3):459–75.
12. Dadfarmay S, Berkowitz R, Kim B, et al. Differentiating pulmonary arterial and pulmonary venous hypertension and the implications for therapy. Congest Heart Fail 2010;16(6):287–91.
13. Fauzi A. Primary pulmonary hypertension. Med J Malaysia 2000;55(4):529–37 [quiz: 538].
14. Proceedings of the 3rd World Symposium on Pulmonary Arterial Hypertension (Venice, Italy) June 23-25, 2003. J Am Coll Cardiol 2004;43:S1–90.
15. Hsu VM, Moreyra AE, Wilson AC, et al. Assessment of pulmonary arterial hypertension in patients with systemic sclerosis: comparison of noninvasive tests with results of right-heart catheterization. J Rheumatol 2008;35(3):458–65.
16. Simonneau G, Robbins IM, Beghetti M, et al. Updated clinical classification of pulmonary hypertension. J Am Coll Cardiol 2009;54(Suppl 1):S43–54.
17. Gurubhagavatula I, Palevsky HI. Pulmonary hypertension in systemic autoimmune disease. Rheum Dis Clin North Am 1997;23(2):365–94.
18. Chemla D, Castelain V, Herve P, et al. Haemodynamic evaluation of pulmonary hypertension. Eur Respir J 2002;20(5):1314–31.
19. Humbert M, Morrell NW, Archer SL, et al. Cellular and molecular pathobiology of pulmonary arterial hypertension. J Am Coll Cardiol 2004;43(12 Suppl S): 13S–24S.

20. Lim KA, Kim KC, Cho MS, et al. Gene expression of endothelin-1 and endothelin receptor a on monocrotaline-induced pulmonary hypertension in rats after bosentan treatment. Korean Circ J 2010;40(9):459–64.
21. Chen CN, Watson G, Zhao L. Cyclic guanosine monophosphate signalling pathway in pulmonary arterial hypertension. Vascul Pharmacol 2012;58(3):211–8.
22. Mahowald ML, Weir EK, Ridley DJ, et al. Pulmonary hypertension in systemic lupus erythematosus: effect of vasodilators on pulmonary hemodynamics. J Rheumatol 1985;12(4):773–7.
23. Jonigk D, Golpon H, Bockmeyer CL, et al. Plexiform lesions in pulmonary arterial hypertension composition, architecture, and microenvironment. Am J Pathol 2011;179(1):167–79.
24. Austin E, Lahm T, West J, et al. Gender, sex hormones and pulmonary hypertension. Pulm Circ 2013;3(2):294–314.
25. Rich S, Dantzker DR, Ayres SM, et al. Primary pulmonary hypertension. A national prospective study. Ann Intern Med 1987;107(2):216–23.
26. Fagan K. Pulmonary arterial hypertension. In: Hanley M, Welsh C, editors. Current diagnosis and treatment in pulmonary medicine. New York: McGraw-Hill; 2003. Available at: http://www.accessmedicine.com/content.aspx?aID=576600. Accessed July 24, 2013.
27. Palevsky HI. The early diagnosis of pulmonary arterial hypertension: can we do better? Chest 2011;140(1):4–6.
28. Zhang RF, Zhou L, Ma GF, et al. Diagnostic value of transthoracic Doppler echocardiography in pulmonary hypertension: a meta-analysis. Am J Hypertens 2010;23(12):1261–4.
29. Goto K, Arai M, Watanabe A, et al. Utility of echocardiography versus BNP level for the prediction of pulmonary arterial pressure in patients with pulmonary arterial hypertension. Int Heart J 2010;51(5):343–7.
30. Badesch DB, Champion HC, Sanchez MA, et al. Diagnosis and assessment of pulmonary arterial hypertension. J Am Coll Cardiol 2009;54(Suppl 1):S55–66.
31. Celebi Sozener Z, Karabiyikoglu G, Duzgun N. Evaluation of the functional parameters in scleroderma cases with pulmonary involvement. Tuberk Toraks 2010;58(3):235–41.
32. Sanchez O, Marie E, Lerolle U, et al. Pulmonary arterial hypertension in women. Rev Mal Respir 2008;25(4):451–60 [in French].
33. Mathai SC, Sibley CT, Forfia PR, et al. Tricuspid annular plane systolic excursion is a robust outcome measure in systemic sclerosis-associated pulmonary arterial hypertension. J Rheumatol 2011;38(11):2410–8.
34. Saito Y, Nakamura K, Miyaji K, et al. Acute vasoreactivity testing with nicardipine in patients with pulmonary arterial hypertension. J Pharmacol Sci 2012;120(3):206–12.
35. Shimony A, Fox BD, Langleben D, et al. Incidence and significance of pericardial effusion in patients with pulmonary arterial hypertension. Can J Cardiol 2013;29(6):678–82.
36. Eysmann SB, Palevsky HI, Reichek N, et al. Two-dimensional and Doppler-echocardiographic and cardiac catheterization correlates of survival in primary pulmonary hypertension. Circulation 1989;80(2):353–60.
37. Burger C, Zeigler T. What can be learned in 6 minutes? 6-minute walk test: primer and role in pulmonary arterial hypertension. Adv Pulm Hypertens 2010; 9(2):107–11.
38. Impens AJ, Wangkaew S, Seibold JR. The 6-minute walk test in scleroderma—how measuring everything measures nothing. Rheumatology (Oxford) 2008; 47(Suppl 5):v68–9.

39. Wasserman K, Hansen J, Sue D, et al. Principles of exercise testing and inter-pretation. 4th edition. Philadelphia: Lea and Febiger; 2005.
40. Heresi GA, Tang WH, Aytekin M, et al. Sensitive cardiac troponin I predicts poor outcomes in pulmonary arterial hypertension. Eur Respir J 2012;39(4): 939–44.
41. Rhodes CJ, Wharton J, Howard LS, et al. Red cell distribution width outperforms other potential circulating biomarkers in predicting survival in idiopathic pulmonary arterial hypertension. Heart 2011;97(13):1054–60.
42. Cracowski JL, Leuchte HH. The potential of biomarkers in pulmonary arterial hypertension. Am J Cardiol 2012;110(Suppl 6):32S–8S.
43. Hesselstrand R, Scheja A, Wuttge DM, et al. Enlarged right-sided dimensions and fibrosis of the right ventricular insertion point on cardiovascular magnetic resonance imaging is seen early in patients with pulmonary arterial hypertension associated with connective tissue disease. Scand J Rheumatol 2011;40(2): 133–8.
44. Haage P, Piroth W, Krombach G, et al. Pulmonary embolism: comparison of angiography with spiral computed tomography, magnetic resonance angiography, and real-time magnetic resonance imaging. Am J Respir Crit Care Med 2003;167(5):729–34.
45. Nicod P, Moser KM. Primary pulmonary hypertension. The risk and benefit of lung biopsy. Circulation 1989;80(5):1486–8.
46. Prabu A, Patel K, Yee CS, et al. Prevalence and risk factors for pulmonary arterial hypertension in patients with lupus. Rheumatology (Oxford) 2009;48(12): 1506–11.
47. Vachiery JL, Coghlan G. Screening for pulmonary arterial hypertension in systemic sclerosis. Eur Respir Rev 2009;18(113):162–9.
48. Rajaram S, Swift AJ, Capener D, et al. Comparison of the diagnostic utility of cardiac magnetic resonance imaging, computed tomography, and echocardiography in assessment of suspected pulmonary arterial hypertension in patients with connective tissue disease. J Rheumatol 2012;39(6):1265–74.
49. Morrell NW, Adnot S, Archer SL, et al. Cellular and molecular basis of pulmonary arterial hypertension. J Am Coll Cardiol 2009;54(Suppl 1):S20–31.
50. Proudman SM, Stevens WM, Sahhar J, et al. Pulmonary arterial hypertension in systemic sclerosis: the need for early detection and treatment. Intern Med J 2007;37(7):485–94.
51. Chung L, Liu J, Parsons L, et al. Characterization of connective tissue disease-associated pulmonary arterial hypertension from REVEAL: identifying systemic sclerosis as a unique phenotype. Chest 2010;138(6):1383–94.
52. Callejas-Rubio JL, Moreno-Escobar E, de la Fuente PM, et al. Prevalence of exercise pulmonary arterial hypertension in scleroderma. J Rheumatol 2008;35(9): 1812–6.
53. Bijl M, Bootsma H, Kallenberg CG. Pulmonary arterial hypertension in systemic lupus erythematosus: should we bother? Rheumatology (Oxford) 2009;48(12): 1471–2.
54. Koh ET, Lee P, Gladman DD, et al. Pulmonary hypertension in systemic sclerosis: an analysis of 17 patients. Br J Rheumatol 1996;35(10):989–93.
55. Campo A, Mathai SC, Le Pavec J, et al. Hemodynamic predictors of survival in scleroderma-related pulmonary arterial hypertension. Am J Respir Crit Care Med 2010;182(2):252–60.
56. Hassoun PM. Therapies for scleroderma-related pulmonary arterial hypertension. Expert Rev Respir Med 2009;3(2):187–96.

57. van Laar JM, Stolk J, Tyndall A. Scleroderma lung: pathogenesis, evaluation and current therapy. Drugs 2007;67(7):985–96.
58. Carmier D, Marchand-Adam S, Diot P, et al. Respiratory involvement in systemic lupus erythematosus. Rev Mal Respir 2008;25(10):1289–303.
59. Guillevin L. Vasculopathy and pulmonary arterial hypertension. Rheumatology (Oxford) 2009;48(Suppl 3):iii54–7.
60. Launay D, Hachulla E, Hatron PY, et al. Pulmonary arterial hypertension: a rare complication of primary Sjogren syndrome: report of 9 new cases and review of the literature. Medicine 2007;86(5):299–315.
61. Tillie-Leblond I, Colin G, Lelong J, et al. Pulmonary involvement in polymyositis and dermatomyositis. Rev Mal Respir 2006;23(6):671–80 [in French].
62. Nagasaka J, Harigai M, Tateis M, et al. Efficacy of combination treatment with cyclosporin A and corticosteroids for acute interstitial pneumonitis associated with dermatomyositis. Mod Rheumatol 2003;13:231–8.
63. Benedict N, Seybert A, Mathier MA. Evidence-based pharmacologic management of pulmonary arterial hypertension. Clin Ther 2007;29(10):2134–53.
64. Oudiz RJ, Schilz RJ, Barst RJ, et al. Treprostinil, a prostacyclin analogue, in pulmonary arterial hypertension associated with connective tissue disease. Chest 2004;126(2):420–7.
65. Frumkin LR. The pharmacological treatment of pulmonary arterial hypertension. Pharmacol Rev 2012;64(3):583–620.
66. Mathai SC, Hassoun PM. Therapy for pulmonary arterial hypertension associated with systemic sclerosis. Curr Opin Rheumatol 2009;21(6):642–8.
67. Galie N, Seeger W, Naeije R, et al. Comparative analysis of clinical trials and evidence-based treatment algorithm in pulmonary arterial hypertension. J Am Coll Cardiol 2004;43(12 Suppl S):81S–8S.
68. Humbert M, Sitbon O, Simonneau G. Treatment of pulmonary arterial hypertension. N Engl J Med 2004;351(14):1425–36.
69. Porhownik N, Al Sharif H, Bshouty Z. Addition of sildenafil in patients with pulmonary arterial hypertension and inadequate response to bosentan monotherapy. Can Respir J 2008;15(8):427–30.
70. McLaughlin V, Humbert M, Coghlan G, et al. Pulmonary arterial hypertension: the most devastating vascular complication of systemic sclerosis. Rheumatology (Oxford) 2009;48(Suppl 3):iii25–31.
71. Vachiery JL. Prostacyclins in pulmonary arterial hypertension: the need for earlier therapy. Adv Ther 2011;28(4):251–69.
72. Nadler ST, Edelman JD. Inhaled treprostinil and pulmonary arterial hypertension. Vasc Health Risk Manag 2010;6:1115–24.
73. Schachna L, Wigley FM. Targeting mediators of vascular injury in scleroderma. Curr Opin Rheumatol 2002;14(6):686–93.
74. Badesch DB, McLaughlin VV, Delcroix M, et al. Prostanoid therapy for pulmonary arterial hypertension. J Am Coll Cardiol 2004;43(12 Suppl S): 56S–61S.
75. Simonneau G, Torbicki A, Hoeper MM, et al. Selexipag: an oral, selective prostacyclin receptor agonist for the treatment of pulmonary arterial hypertension. Eur Respir J 2012;40(4):874–80.
76. Badesch DB, Abman SH, Ahearn GS, et al. Medical therapy for pulmonary arterial hypertension: ACCP evidence-based clinical practice guidelines. Chest 2004;126(Suppl 1):35S–62S.
77. Barst RJ, Rubin LJ, Long WA, et al, The Primary Pulmonary Hypertension Study Group. A comparison of continuous intravenous epoprostenol (prostacyclin)

with conventional therapy for primary pulmonary hypertension. N Engl J Med 1996;334(5):296–302.

78. Barst RJ, Rubin LJ, McGoon MD, et al. Survival in primary pulmonary hypertension with long-term continuous intravenous prostacyclin. Ann Intern Med 1994; 121(6):409–15.

79. Shapiro SM, Oudiz RJ, Cao T, et al. Primary pulmonary hypertension: improved long-term effects and survival with continuous intravenous epoprostenol infusion. J Am Coll Cardiol 1997;30(2):343–9.

80. McLaughlin VV, Genthner DE, Panella MM, et al. Reduction in pulmonary vascular resistance with long-term epoprostenol (prostacyclin) therapy in primary pulmonary hypertension. N Engl J Med 1998;338(5):273–7.

81. McLaughlin VV, Shillington A, Rich S. Survival in primary pulmonary hypertension: the impact of epoprostenol therapy. Circulation 2002;106(12):1477–82.

82. Sitbon O, Humbert M, Nunes H, et al. Long-term intravenous epoprostenol infusion in primary pulmonary hypertension: prognostic factors and survival. J Am Coll Cardiol 2002;40(4):780–8.

83. Humbert M, Sanchez O, Fartoukh M, et al. Short-term and long-term epoprostenol (prostacyclin) therapy in pulmonary hypertension secondary to connective tissue diseases: results of a pilot study. Eur Respir J 1999; 13(6):1351–6.

84. Badesch DB, McGoon MD, Barst RJ, et al. Long-term survival among patients with scleroderma-associated pulmonary arterial hypertension treated with intravenous epoprostenol. J Rheumatol 2009;36(10):2244–9.

85. Gaine SP, Rubin LJ. Medical and surgical treatment options for pulmonary hypertension. Am J Med Sci 1998;315(3):179–84.

86. Rubin LJ. Primary pulmonary hypertension. N Engl J Med 1997;336(2):111–7.

87. Yanagisawa M, Kurihara H, Kimura S, et al. A novel potent vasoconstrictor peptide produced by vascular endothelial cells. Nature 1988;332(6163): 411–5.

88. Dupuis J, Stewart DJ, Cernacek P, et al. Human pulmonary circulation is an important site for both clearance and production of endothelin-1. Circulation 1996;94(7):1578–84.

89. Channick RN, Simonneau G, Sitbon O, et al. Effects of the dual endothelin-receptor antagonist bosentan in patients with pulmonary hypertension: a randomised placebo-controlled study. Lancet 2001;358(9288):1119–23.

90. Rubin LJ, Badesch DB, Barst RJ, et al. Bosentan therapy for pulmonary arterial hypertension. N Engl J Med 2002;346(12):896–903.

91. Galie N, Rubin L, Hoeper M, et al. Treatment of patients with mildly symptomatic pulmonary arterial hypertension with bosentan (EARLY study): a double-blind, randomised controlled trial. Lancet 2008;371(9630):2093–100.

92. Galie N, Olschewski H, Oudiz RJ, et al. Ambrisentan for the treatment of pulmonary arterial hypertension: results of the ambrisentan in pulmonary arterial hypertension, randomized, double-blind, placebo-controlled, multicenter, efficacy (ARIES) study 1 and 2. Circulation 2008;117(23):3010–9.

93. Bolli MH, Boss C, Binkert C, et al. The discovery of N-[5-(4-bromophenyl)-6-[2-[(5-bromo-2-pyrimidinyl)oxy]ethoxy]-4-pyrimidinyl]-N'-p ropylsulfamide (Macitentan), an orally active, potent dual endothelin receptor antagonist. J Med Chem 2012;55(17):7849–61.

94. Mikhail GW, Prasad SK, Li W, et al. Clinical and haemodynamic effects of sildenafil in pulmonary hypertension: acute and mid-term effects. Eur Heart J 2004; 25(5):431–6.

95. Michelakis E, Tymchak W, Lien D, et al. Oral sildenafil is an effective and specific pulmonary vasodilator in patients with pulmonary arterial hypertension: comparison with inhaled nitric oxide. Circulation 2002;105(20):2398–403.
96. Galie N, Ghofrani HA, Torbicki A, et al. Sildenafil citrate therapy for pulmonary arterial hypertension. N Engl J Med 2005;353(20):2148–57.
97. Zhao L, Mason NA, Morrell NW, et al. Sildenafil inhibits hypoxia-induced pulmonary hypertension. Circulation 2001;104(4):424–8.
98. Sastry BK, Narasimhan C, Reddy NK, et al. Clinical efficacy of sildenafil in primary pulmonary hypertension: a randomized, placebo-controlled, double-blind, crossover study. J Am Coll Cardiol 2004;43(7):1149–53.
99. Wilkins MR, Paul GA, Strange JW, et al. Sildenafil versus endothelin receptor antagonist for pulmonary hypertension (SERAPH) study. Am J Respir Crit Care Med 2005;171(11):1292–7.
100. Badesch DB, Hill NS, Burgess G, et al. Sildenafil for pulmonary arterial hypertension associated with connective tissue disease. J Rheumatol 2007;34(12):2417–22.
101. Levin YD, White RJ. Novel therapeutic approaches in pulmonary arterial hypertension: focus on tadalafil. Drugs Today (Barc) 2011;47(2):145–56.
102. Falk JA, Philip KJ, Schwarz ER. The emergence of oral tadalafil as a once-daily treatment for pulmonary arterial hypertension. Vasc Health Risk Manag 2010;6:273–80.
103. Oudiz RJ, Brundage BH, Galie N, et al. Tadalafil for the treatment of pulmonary arterial hypertension: a double-blind 52-week uncontrolled extension study. J Am Coll Cardiol 2012;60(8):768–74.
104. Grimminger F, Schermuly RT, Ghofrani HA. Targeting non-malignant disorders with tyrosine kinase inhibitors. Nat Rev Drug Discov 2010;9(12):956–70.
105. Sakao S, Tatsumi K. Vascular remodeling in pulmonary arterial hypertension: multiple cancer-like pathways and possible treatment modalities. Int J Cardiol 2011;147(1):4–12.
106. Ghofrani HA, Morrell NW, Hoeper MM, et al. Imatinib in pulmonary arterial hypertension patients with inadequate response to established therapy. Am J Respir Crit Care Med 2010;182(9):1171–7.
107. Song KW, Rifkind J, Al-Beirouti B, et al. Subdural hematomas during CML therapy with imatinib mesylate. Leuk Lymphoma 2004;45(8):1633–6.
108. Patel SB, Gojo I, Tidwell ML, et al. Subdural hematomas in patients with Philadelphia chromosome-positive acute lymphoblastic leukemia receiving imatinib mesylate in conjunction with systemic and intrathecal chemotherapy. Leuk Lymphoma 2011;52(7):1211–4.
109. Michelakis ED. Soluble guanylate cyclase stimulators as a potential therapy for PAH: enthusiasm, pragmatism and concern. Eur Respir J 2009;33(4):717–21.
110. Schermuly RT, Janssen W, Weissmann N, et al. Riociguat for the treatment of pulmonary hypertension. Expert Opin Investig Drugs 2011;20(4):567–76.
111. Ghofrani H, Galie N, Grimminger F, et al. Riociguat for the treatment of pulmonary arterial hypertension. N Engl J Med 2013;369:330–40.
112. Mittendorf J, Weigand S, Alonso-Alija C, et al. Discovery of riociguat (BAY 63-2521): a potent, oral stimulator of soluble guanylate cyclase for the treatment of pulmonary hypertension. ChemMedChem 2009;4(5):853–65.
113. Gentile MA. Inhaled medical gases: more to breathe than oxygen. Respir Care 2011;56(9):1341–57 [discussion: 1357–49].
114. Hoeper MM, Markevych I, Spiekerkoetter E, et al. Goal-oriented treatment and combination therapy for pulmonary arterial hypertension. Eur Respir J 2005;26(5):858–63.

115. Kemp K, Savale L, O'Callaghan DS, et al. Usefulness of first-line combination therapy with epoprostenol and bosentan in pulmonary arterial hypertension: an observational study. J Heart Lung Transplant 2012;31(2):150–8.

116. Simonneau G, Rubin LJ, Galie N, et al. Addition of sildenafil to long-term intravenous epoprostenol therapy in patients with pulmonary arterial hypertension: a randomized trial. Ann Intern Med 2008;149(8):521–30.

117. Fox BD, Shimony A, Langleben D. Meta-analysis of monotherapy versus combination therapy for pulmonary arterial hypertension. Am J Cardiol 2011;108(8): 1177–82.

118. Humbert M, Barst RJ, Robbins IM, et al. Combination of bosentan with epoprostenol in pulmonary arterial hypertension: BREATHE-2. Eur Respir J 2004;24(3): 353–9.

119. McLaughlin VV, Benza RL, Rubin LJ, et al. Addition of inhaled treprostinil to oral therapy for pulmonary arterial hypertension: a randomized controlled clinical trial. J Am Coll Cardiol 2010;55(18):1915–22.

120. Lordan JL, Corris PA. Pulmonary arterial hypertension and lung transplantation. Expert Rev Respir Med 2011;5(3):441–54.

121. Long J, Russo MJ, Muller C, et al. Surgical treatment of pulmonary hypertension: lung transplantation. Pulm Circ 2011;1(3):327–33.

122. Kamler M, Pizanis N, Aleksic I, et al. Pulmonary hypertension and lung transplantation. Herz 2005;30(4):281–5 [in German].

123. Levine SM, Anzueto A, Peters JI, et al. Single lung transplantation in patients with systemic disease. Chest 1994;105(3):837–41.

124. Pigula FA, Griffith BP, Zenati MA, et al. Lung transplantation for respiratory failure resulting from systemic disease. Ann Thorac Surg 1997;64(6):1630–4.

125. Rosas V, Conte JV, Yang SC, et al. Lung transplantation and systemic sclerosis. Ann Transplant 2000;5(3):38–43.

126. Denton CP, Hachulla E. Risk factors associated with pulmonary arterial hypertension in patients with systemic sclerosis and implications for screening. Eur Respir Rev 2011;20(122):270–6.

127. Condliffe R, Kiely DG, Peacock AJ, et al. Connective tissue disease-associated pulmonary arterial hypertension in the modern treatment era. Am J Respir Crit Care Med 2009;179(2):151–7.

128. Benza RL, Miller DP, Barst RJ, et al. An evaluation of long-term survival from time of diagnosis in pulmonary arterial hypertension from the REVEAL Registry. Chest 2012;142(2):448–56.

129. Kovacs G, Maier R, Aberer E, et al. Pulmonary arterial hypertension therapy may be safe and effective in patients with systemic sclerosis and borderline pulmonary artery pressure. Arthritis Rheum 2012;64(4):1257–62.

130. Olschewski H. Pulmonary hypertension: the future has begun. Med Klin (Munich) 2006;101(4):328–33.

131. Agarwal R, Gomberg-Maitland M. Current therapeutics and practical management strategies for pulmonary arterial hypertension. Am Heart J 2011;162(2): 201–13.

Gout and the Heart

Vidula Bhole, MD[a], Eswar Krishnan, MD, M.Phil[b],*

KEYWORDS

- Gout • Uric acid • Risk cardiovascular • Coronary • Mortality

KEY POINTS

- Gout is associated with higher risk of cardiovascular events in almost all the published studies.
- Patients with gout undergoing medical therapy are statistically less likely to have cardiovascular disease (CVD) than those not undergoing therapy.
- The relative importance of anti-inflammatory therapies and urate-lowering therapies in potentially reducing the CVD risk is under intense investigation.

"The gout has treated me with more severity than any former time; it however never climbed higher than my ankles."
—British author and poet Samuel Johnson (1709–1784)

Unfortunately, gout is known to climb much higher than ankles; the heart is the most important organ affected.

INTRODUCTION

Humans are distinguished from other mammals by the absence of serum uricase, a hepatic enzyme that converts uric acid to allantoin; the latter is soluble in water and readily excreted. The absence of uricase along with extensive reabsorption of uric acid in the proximal tubules of kidney results in tenfold higher levels of serum uric acid in humans than in other mammals.[1] Serum uric acid may act as antioxidant, thus providing some protection against aging and cancer.[2] In some individuals, however, serum uric acid levels are higher than normal; this condition is defined as hyperuricemia. For epidemiologic studies, Krishnan and colleagues[3] defined hyperuricemia as a serum uric acid concentration greater than 7.0 mg/dL. Serum uric acid levels in premenopausal women are lower by about 1 mg/dL than in men, owing to higher renal

Disclosures: Dr E. Krishnan has received honoraria, consultation fees, and research grants from the following entities in the past 3 years: Takeda, Metabolex, Savient, ARDEA (Currently owned by Astra Zeneca). Dr V. Bhole has no disclosures to declare.
[a] 515 Olmsted Road, Palo Alto, CA 94305, USA; [b] ARAMIS Program, Department of Medicine, Stanford University, 1000 Welch Road, Suite 203, Palo Alto, CA 94304, USA
* Corresponding author.
E-mail address: e.krishnan@stanford.edu

clearance of urate in women, possibly due to their higher plasma estrogen levels.[4] Therefore, it can be argued that definitions of hyperuricemia should differ based on gender. Therefore, hyperuricemia is also defined as a uric acid level greater than 7.0 mg/dL in men and greater than 5.7 mg/dL in women.[5] Hyperuricemia may lead to gout and nephrolithiasis, although whether to treat subjects with asymptomatic hyperuricemia is debatable. Large population-based studies have shown that the incidence of gout increases with increasing serum uric acid levels.[6] Gout is a common and excruciatingly painful inflammatory arthritis, characterized by recurrent attacks of acute arthritis due to the crystallization of monosodium urate within joints. In some patients, gout leads to development of chronic arthritis and urate tophi.

Galen, a Roman physician of the second century, astutely stated that gout is due to a "hereditary trait" and to "debauchery and intemperance." The association between gout and cardiovascular disease (CVD) was also observed in Roman times. In the 19th century, physicians in England and elsewhere noted that people with gout tend to die from other causes earlier in life.[7,8] In the 1950s, one of the founding objectives of the Framingham heart study was to test the hypothesis that gout is associated with coronary artery disease.[9] The first modern article linking gout and unstable angina was published in 1988 and was based on data from the Framingham study.[10] More recently, the focus has been on the association between hyperuricemia and CVD. Convincing cross-sectional associations have been reported linking progressive increase in serum uric acid with greater coronary artery calcifications (**Figs. 1** and **2**). Prospective studies have demonstrated strong independent associations between serum urate concentrations and incidence of hypertension and incidence of heart failure (**Figs. 3** and **4**). Over the past decade, there has been a resurgence of interest in the association between gout and heart disease driven by emerging epidemiologic data linking the two, the realization that gouty arthritis and hyperuricemia are not synonymous but distinct pathophysiologic entities, and that the inflammatory activity in gout may provide additional risk for CVD. This article focuses on the epidemiologic associations of gout with MI and CAD (collectively referred as CVD here) and with heart failure.

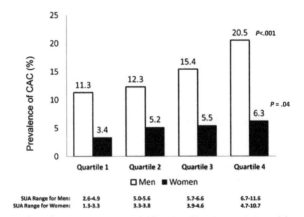

Fig. 1. Prevalence of any coronary artery calcification (Agatston score >0) by serum uric acid concentration among participants (1211 men and 1287 women) in the Coronary Artery Risk Development in Young Adults (CARDIA) study cohort at year 15. *P* values are for trend test. CAC, coronary artery calcification; SUA, serum urate. (*From* Krishnan E, Pandya BJ, Chung L, et al. Hyperuricemia and the risk for subclinical coronary atherosclerosis–data from a prospective observational cohort study. Arthritis Res Ther 2011;13(2):R66.)

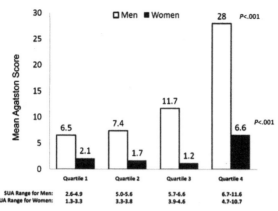

Fig. 2. Relationship between burden of coronary artery calcification (unmodified Agatston score) and serum uric acid (SUA) concentrations among 238 subjects in the CARDIA study cohort who had an Agatston score of greater than zero. *P* values are for trend test. (*From* Krishnan E, Pandya BJ, Chung L, et al. Hyperuricemia and the risk for subclinical coronary atherosclerosis—data from a prospective observational cohort study. Arthritis Res Ther 2011;13(2):R66.)

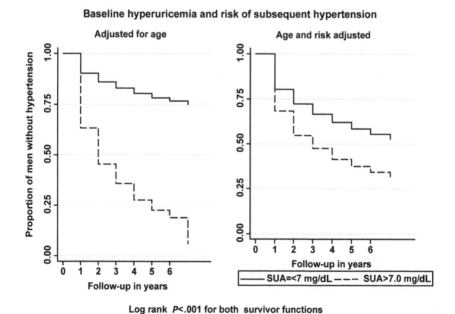

Fig. 3. Time to develop hypertension among 803 men in the Multiple Risk Factor Intervention Trial (MRFIT) without metabolic syndrome but with baseline hyperuricemia (serum uric acid [SUA] >7.0 mg/dL) compared with 2270 men without hyperuricemia, adjusted for baseline values of age, systolic and diastolic blood pressure, serum creatinine, proteinuria, serum triglycerides, total cholesterol, alcohol use, smoking, and BMI. (*From* Krishnan E, Kwoh CK, Schumacher HR, et al. Hyperuricemia and incidence of hypertension among men without metabolic syndrome. Hypertension 2007;49(2):298–303.)

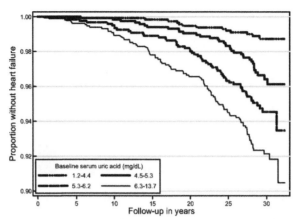

Fig. 4. Kaplan-Meier estimates for heart failure–free follow-up among the 4912 participants of the Framingham Offspring Study by quartiles of serum uric acid. For this survival model, the observation started at the first study visit and ended at the time of incident heart failure (n = 196). The y-axis scale is adjusted for the sake of clarity. (*From* Krishnan E. Hyperuricemia and incident heart failure. Circ Heart Fail 2009;2(6):559; with permission.)

ASSOCIATION BETWEEN GOUT AND CVD
Case Series and Cross-sectional Studies

In general, case-series and cross-sectional studies are considered less valuable than cohort studies in establishing causality. Nevertheless, these studies are easier to perform, less expensive, provide important insights and corroborating data with respect to the association between gout and coronary artery disease, and have paved the path for future research. **Table 1** summarizes the key studies of this type that have assessed associations between gout and CVD.

The earliest case series to report associations between gout and CVD mortality were published in the 1980s, but they were without comparative populations.[11,12] In a large-scale cross-sectional study, Chen and colleagues[13] evaluated whether the severity of gouty arthritis is associated with Q-wave myocardial infarction (QWMI). In multivariate analyses controlling for serum urate level, age, gender, smoking, drinking, diuretics use, total cholesterol, triglyceride, hypertension, diabetes, and body mass index (BMI), they found that increased affected joint count was associated with QWMI. A recent study from New Zealand showed that participants with gout were more likely to have cardiac disease history (defined as history of angina, myocardial infarction [MI], heart failure, stroke, cardiac intervention, pacemaker, percutaneous transluminal coronary angioplasty, coronary artery bypass graft surgery, or other cardiac intervention). About 17.5% of individuals with gout had cardiac history compared with only 3.5% without gout. The difference was significant after adjusting for age and gender.[14] Another study conducted in New Zealand adults using administrative data showed that CVD is more prevalent in subjects with gout, compared with those without gout.[15]

Case-control and Cohort Studies

In observational epidemiologic research, case-control studies, case-control studies nested in a cohort, and cohort studies are used to establish causality. Prospectively collected data, with minimal attrition, provides a wealth of information. Knowledge of the association between gout and CVD comes from data collected prospectively

Table 1
Major case-series and cross-sectional studies of gout and CVD

Study (Ref.)	Subject Source	Number of Subjects Gout (Total)	Follow-up Years[a]	CVD Outcomes	Number of subjects with CVD outcomes, Gout (Total)	Adjusted Effect Size (95% CI)
Yü et al,[11] 1980 (USA)	Research clinic case series	2000	30	Mortality	382	N/A (descriptive data)
Nishioka & Mikanagi,[12] 1981 (Japan)	Clinics case series	104	8	CVD	28	N/A (descriptive data)
Darlington et al,[51] 1983 (UK)	Clinics	180	6	CVD mortality	5	N/A (O/E, gout not significant)
Chen et al,[13] 2007 (Taiwan)	Administrative data	22,572	N/A	Q waves in ECG	393	1.18 (1.01–1.38); gout significant
Stamp et al,[14] 2013 (New Zealand)	Population	57 (751)	N/A	CVD by history	10 (24)	Significant difference
Winnard et al,[15] 2011 (New Zealand)	Administrative data	119,234 (3,036,093)	N/A	CVD	27,131 (165,042)	Age-standardized rate ratio 2.7 (P<.001)

Abbreviations: CHD, coronary heart disease; MI, myocardial infarction; O/E: ratio of observed versus expected deaths.

[a] Follow-up years are the maximum number of years if given as a single number. If given in mean (SD) format then mean follow-up and standard deviation for that study is shown.

Data from Refs.[11–15,51]

over the last several decades. The major cohort studies that have evaluated the association between fatal and nonfatal coronary artery disease and gout are summarized in **Table 2**; see later discussion.

In one of the first nested case-control studies to evaluate the association between gout and CVD, De Muckadell and Gyntelberg[16] compared Copenhagen men 40 to 59 years old with (104) and without (208) gout. They found that angina pectoris occurred more frequently among the gout cases than among controls (11.5% vs 2.4%, $P<.001$) but observed no significant differences in the occurrence of MI. The earliest large-scale cohort study published in English that documented the association between gout and CVD was published in 1988. Abbott and colleagues[10] analyzed Framingham Heart Study data to study the association between gout without the use of diuretics and risk of coronary heart disease (CHD). Men with gout experienced a 60% excess of CHD and 80% increased risk of angina pectoris compared with those without gout; the association was significant after adjusting for age, systolic blood pressure, total cholesterol, alcohol, BMI, and diabetes. For women, no significant associations were observed. Major limitations of this study were an insufficient number of individuals with gout and unclear validity of self-report of gout. Furthermore, the investigators did not account for confounding by major factors, including uric acid, smoking, and renal function.

The data from the Meharry and Johns Hopkins Precursors cohorts of male physicians were used by Gelber and colleagues[17] to study the association of gout and CVD risk. There were very few outcome events in individuals with gout: only three CHD events among the 31 subjects in the gout group in the Meharry cohort and four events in the group of 62 subjects with gout in the Johns Hopkins Precursors cohort. Among 1446 subjects without gout, 175 events occurred in both cohorts combined. The pooled, risk-adjusted relative risk (RR) was 0.59, with a wide CI (0.24–1.46). The direction of risk is counterintuitive and may be accounted for unresolved confounding and interaction in their analyses by measures of renal function, and use of aspirin and diuretics. Renal function, use of diuretics, and serum uric acid levels were not considered in the analyses.

Two other large-scale studies on gout and heart disease were based on the Multiple Risk Factor Intervention Trial (MRFIT).[3,18] The MRFIT was a randomized controlled trial designed to examine the efficacy of a program of coronary risk reduction among men at high risk of adverse coronary events. Overall, 12,866 men in the MRFIT were followed up for a mean of 6.5 years. Krishnan and colleagues[3] assessed whether gouty arthritis was a risk factor for acute MI in the MRFIT cohort, independent of renal function, diuretic use, metabolic syndrome, and other established risk factors. Using multivariable logistic regression adjusted for these risk factors, they found that gout was associated with 26% higher risk of acute MI (odds ratio [OR] 1.26; 95% CI 1.14–1.40). The association persisted among nonusers of alcohol, diuretics, or aspirin, and among subjects who did not have metabolic syndrome, diabetes mellitus, or obesity. Furthermore, a relationship between gout and the risk of acute MI was evident among subjects with and without hyperuricemia. In the second study using the MRFIT data, associations of gout with CVD, MI, and CHD death were examined.[18] Cox proportional hazards regression analysis was used and multivariable models were adjusted for age, systolic and diastolic blood pressure, low-density and high-density lipoprotein cholesterol levels, plasma triglyceride levels, serum creatinine levels, fasting glucose levels, cigarettes and alcoholic drinks per day, family history of MI assessed at baseline, daily aspirin and diuretic use, and BMI. The unadjusted mortality rates from CVD among subjects with and without gout were 10.3 per 1000 person-years and 8.0 per 1000 person-years, respectively,

Table 2
Major cohort and nested case-control studies of gout and CVD

Study (Ref.)	Population	Number of Subjects Gout (Total)	Follow-up Years[a]	Outcomes	Number of Subjects with CHD Outcome (Total Number of Cases of Gout)	Adjusted Effect Size (95% CI)[b]
Abbott et al,[10] 1988 (USA)	Framingham cohort[c]	94 (1858)	32	CHD	37 (509)	1.60 (1.10–2.50); significant
Gelber et al,[17] 1997 (USA)	Meharry-Hopkins cohort	93 (1624)	30	CHD	7 (182)	0.59 (0.24–1.46); not significant
Janssens et al,[52] 2003 (Netherlands)	Continuous Morbidity Registration cohort	170 (510)	11	CVD	44 (114)	0.98 (0.65–1.47); not significant
Krishnan et al,[3] 2006 (USA)	Multiple Risk Factor Intervention Trial cohort	1123 (12,866)	6.5	Fatal MI / All MI	22 (246) / 118 (1108)	0.96 (0.66–1.44); not significant / 1.26 (1.14–1.40); significant
Choi & Curhan,[19] 2007 (USA)	Health Professionals Follow-up cohort	2773 (51,297)	12	CVD mortality / CHD mortality / Nonfatal MI	304 (2132) / 238 (1576) / 23 (1152)	1.38 (1.15–1.66); significant / 1.55 (1.24–1.93); significant / 1.59 (1.04–2.41); significant
Krishnan et al,[18] 2008 (USA)	MRFIT cohort	655 (9105)	17	Fatal MI / CHD mortality / CVD mortality	36 (360) / 78 (833) / 110 (1241)	1.35 (0.94–1.93); not significant / 1.35 (1.06–1.72); significant / 1.21 (0.99–1.49); not significant
Cohen et al,[53] 2008 (USA)	US Renal Data System dialysis subjects	24,415 (234,794)	5	CVD mortality	Not reported	1.47 (1.26–1.59); significant
Kuo et al,[22] 2010 (Taiwan)	Participants of a health-screening program conducted by the Chang Gung Memorial Hospital in Taiwan (2000–2006)	1311 (61,527)	4.7 (2)	CVD mortality	12 (198)	1.97 (1.08–3.59); significant

(continued on next page)

Table 2
(continued)

Study (Ref.)	Population	Number of Subjects Gout (Total)	Follow-up Years[a]	Outcomes	Number of Subjects with CHD Outcome (Total Number of Cases of Gout)	Adjusted Effect Size (95% CI)[b]
De Vera et al,[20] 2010 (Canada)	Case and control cohorts selected from British Columbia (Canada) Musculoskeletal Cohort: 3.5 million subjects with any musculoskeletal diagnosis between 1991 and 2004	Men and women together: 9642 (57,852) Only women: 3890 (23,340)	10	Women All MI	244 (996)	Women 1.39 (1.20–1.61); significant
				Fatal MI	61 (261)	1.33 (0.99–1.78); not significant
				Nonfatal MI	183 (735)	1.41 (1.19–1.67); significant
				Men All MI	435 (2272)	Men 1.11 (0.99–1.23); not significant
				Fatal MI	100 (517)	1.10 (0.88–1.38); not significant
				Nonfatal MI	335 (1755)	1.11 (0.98–1.25); not significant
Teng et al,[21] 2012 (Singapore)	The Singapore Chinese Health Study, a population-based, prospective study of Chinese individuals in Singapore, 45–74 y at recruitment (1993–1998)	2117 (52,322)	8.1 (mean)	CHD deaths	85 (1213)	1.38 (1.10–1.73); significant

Study	Cohort/Database	No. with gout (No. without gout)	Follow-up (y)	Outcome	No. of events	Hazard ratio (95% CI); significance
Kok et al,[23] 2012 (Taiwan)	Taiwan National Health Insurance Research Database, nondiabetic >50 y	164,463 (3,694,377)	4	CVD mortality	5650 (74,367)	1.10 (1.07–1.13); significant
Kuo et al,[54] 2013 (Taiwan)	Taiwan National Health Insurance database	26,556 (704,503)	9	All MI	463 (3718)	1.23 (1.11–1.36); significant
				Fatal MI	35 (299)	0.97 (0.68–1.39); not significant
				Nonfatal MI	428 (3419)	1.26 (1.14–1.40); significant
				Individuals without cardiovascular risk factors all MIs	112 (1739)	1.84 (1.51–2.24); significant
				Individuals without cardiovascular risk factors nonfatal MIs	Not available	1.80 (1.49–3.95); significant
Stack et al,[24] 2013 (USA)	NHANES III cohort	— (15,773)	10	Cardiovascular mortality	— (1276)	1.46 (1.07–2.00); significant

Abbreviation: CHD, coronary heart disease.

[a] Follow-up years are the maximum number of years if given as a single number. If given in mean (SD) format then mean follow-up and standard deviation for that study is shown.

[b] Significant or not significant indicates whether or not gout is an independent predictor of outcome.

[c] Results reported for men only.

Data from Refs.[3,10,17–24,53,54]

representing an approximately 30% greater risk for CVD in subjects with gout compared with those without gout. One major limitation of both these studies was that men in the MRFIT study group were at high risk for CHD. Although gout was self-reported, which is a limitation, the investigators added the requirement of sustained hyperuricemia (serum uric acid of $\geq$7.0 mg/dL).

In another larger observational study, Choi and Curhan[19] prospectively examined the relation between a history of gout and the risk of death and MI in 51,297 male participants of the Health Professionals Follow-Up Study. The extensively adjusted multivariate models (adjusted for age, history of hypertension, hypercholesterolemia, diabetes mellitus, use of aspirin and diuretics, smoking, BMI, physical activity, alcohol intake, family history of MI, and diet) showed an elevated risk of CVD death, particularly from CHD, for subjects with gout. The RRs among men with history of gout were 1.38 (95% CI: 1.15–1.66) for CVD deaths and 1.55 (95% CI: 1.24–1.93) for fatal CHD. The corresponding RRs among men with preexisting CHD were 1.26 (95% CI: 1.07–1.50) and 1.24 (95% CI: 1.04–1.49), respectively. In addition, men with gout had a higher risk of nonfatal MI than men without gout. One major limitation of this study was its restriction to male health professionals, thus affecting generalizability. The use of self-reported gout was another limitation.

In a population-based cohort study of gout cases and controls, De Vera and colleagues[20] found that in multivariate analyses after adjusting for age, comorbidities, and prescription drug use, the risk of acute MI was 39% higher (95% CI: 1.20–1.61) in women with gout and 11% higher (95% CI: 0.99–1.23) in men with gout compared with controls. This study suffered from potential diagnostic misclassification as the diagnostic codes were used to identify gout and MI. The study has significant generalizability because it was population-based. Of particular interest is that women with gout had significantly higher risk of MI than controls did; the magnitude of excess risk was higher than in men with gout.

Recent studies based in Asia have also evaluated associations between gout and CVD. Teng and colleagues[21] assessed the link between gout and CHD mortality in a prospective cohort, the Singapore Chinese Health Study. Individuals in the study were 45 to 74 years old and the study lasted from 1993 to 1998. After a mean follow-up of 8.1 years, subjects with gout had a higher risk of CHD death (multivariable hazard ratio [HR] 1.38; 95% CI: 1.10–1.73) compared with subjects without gout. The association was present in both genders but the risk estimates were higher for women (multivariable HR 1.71; 95% CI: 1.12–2.60). Kuo and colleagues[22] reported the risk of CVD mortality in gout population in Taiwan. The adjusted HR of CVD mortality was almost double in gout subjects compared with normouricemic population (HR 1.97; 95% CI: 1.08–3.59). The major strength of this study was that data were collected from a large sample of community-dwelling adults, both men and women, thus making it generalizable. Moreover, the investigators adjusted for renal function, which previous studies failed to do. A study of individuals in Taiwan by Kok and colleagues[23] found that the multivariable risk for CVD mortality among the individuals with gout was 1.10 (95% CI 1.07–1.13) compared with those without. Interestingly, risk was attenuated in subjects with gout and chronic kidney disease.

Stack and colleagues[24] assessed the association between gout and cardiovascular mortality in the US population using data from the Third National Health and Nutrition Examination Survey (NHANES III). They linked baseline information collected from 1988 to 1994 from NHANES III with mortality data through 2006. The multivariable risk of cardiovascular mortality was increased by 46% in those with gout compared with those without gout (95% CI: 1.07–2.00).

ASSOCIATION BETWEEN GOUT AND CONGESTIVE HEART FAILURE

The association between high levels of urate and heart failure has been demonstrated.[25,26] The studies that have evaluated the association between gout and heart failure are summarized in **Table 3**. Stack and colleagues[24] found that 9.7% (SE 1.8) of individuals in the NHANES III cohort with gout had congestive heart failure (CHF) at baseline compared with 1.8% (SE 0.16) of individuals without gout. A recent study based on NHANES III data from 5707 adult participants (2007–2008) showed that among individuals with gout 11% had heart failure.[27] Based on the analysis of data from the Framingham offspring study, gout is associated with a reduced metrics of cardiac pump function as well as higher incidence of clinical heart failure (**Fig. 5**).[28] In this study, participants with gout had worse metrics of echocardiographic changes signifying myocardial systolic dysfunction (**Table 4**). In the follow-up analyses, mortality was elevated in subgroup of subjects with gout and heart failure (adjusted HR 1.50, 95% CI 1.30–1.73) compared with those with heart failure but without gout (**Table 5**).

Use of anti-gout treatment is associated with better cardiovascular outcomes. Struthers and colleagues[29] examined whether allopurinol was associated with any alteration in mortality and hospitalizations in subjects with CHF in a retrospective cohort study. Using multivariable models, the long-term use of more than 300 mg/day allopurinol was associated with a significantly better mortality than was use of lower doses of allopurinol (RR 0.59; 95% CI 0.37–0.95); numbers of cardiovascular hospitalizations were also reduced in the higher dose cohort (RR 0.49; 95% CI: 0.26–0.91).

Thanassoulis and colleagues[30] conducted nested case-control analysis of healthcare data on a retrospective cohort of 25,090 subjects with symptomatic heart failure who were 66 years or older from Quebec, Canada. Both a remote history of gout and an acute episode of gout (within 60 days of the event date) were associated with an increased risk of heart failure readmission or death (adjusted RR 1.63; 95% CI: 1.48–1.80 and 2.06; 95% CI: 1.39–3.06; respectively). Continuous allopurinol use (>30 days of continuous use) was associated with reduced heart failure readmissions or death (RR = 0.69; 95% CI: 60–0.79) and all-cause mortality (RR = 0.74; 95% CI: 0.61–0.90) among subjects with a history of gout. However, in the overall subject population, there was no statistically significant association between allopurinol use and the combined outcome of heart failure readmission or death (adjusted RR = 1.02; 95% CI: 0.95–1.10; $P = .55$).

ASSOCIATION BETWEEN GOUT AND OTHER CVD RISK FACTORS

Recently Bhole and colleagues[6] analyzed 52 years of follow-up data from the Framingham Heart Study to evaluate risk factors for incident gout among women and to compare them with those among men. The incident rate of gout was much higher in men: 4.0 per 1000 person-years in men compared with 1.4 per 1000 person-years in women. Increasing age, obesity, alcohol consumption, hypertension, and diuretic use were associated with the risk of incident gout. Male gender, age, obesity, alcohol consumption, hypertension, and diuretic use are also risk factors for CVD.

GOUT MEDICATIONS AND CVD OUTCOMES

The available data seem to suggest that patients with gout who are treated with gout medications have CVD outcome rates comparable to nongout individuals, and those not on treatment have significantly higher rates (**Fig. 6**).

Anti-gout medications like xanthine oxidase inhibitors (eg, allopurinol) and colchicine also have cardioprotective effect. This also supports the association between

Table 3
Major studies of gout and heart failure

Study (Ref.)	Population	Study Design	Number of Subjects Gout (Total)	Follow-up Years[a]	Outcomes	Number or % of Subjects with CHD Outcome (Overall)	Adjusted Effect Size (95% CI)[b]
Thanassoulis et al,[30] 2010 (Canada)	General population >65 y with symptomatic heart failure, in Quebec, Canada	Nested case-control in a retrospective cohort	7684 (157,582)	7	Heart failure readmission or death	1053 (14,327)	1.63 (1.48–1.80); significant
Krishnan,[28] 2012 (USA)	Framingham Heart Study Offspring Cohort	Cohort	228 (4519)	37	Incident heart failure Mortality of gout vs no gout among those with heart failure	22 (178)	1.74 (1.03–2.93); significant 1.50 (1.30–1.73); significant
Stack et al,[24] 2013 (USA)	NHANES III cohort (1988–94)	Cross-sectional	—	N/A	Congestive heart failure	9.7 (1.8)	N/A

[a] Follow-up years are the maximum number of years if given as a single number. If given in mean (SD) format then mean follow-up and standard deviation for that study is shown.
[b] Significant or not significant indicates whether or not gout is an independent predictor of outcome.
Data from Refs.[24,28,30]

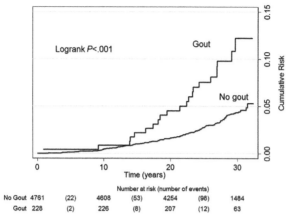

Fig. 5. Nelson-Aalen cumulative risk estimates for heart failure among subjects with and without gout (n = 228 and 4761, respectively) in the Framingham Offspring Study. The number of participants at risk for heart failure in each group is provided in two rows. The number of incident cases of heart failure in each time interval is provided within parenthesis. (*From* Krishnan E. Gout and the risk for incident heart failure and systolic dysfunction. BMJ Open 2012;2(1):e000282.)

Table 4
Echocardiographic characteristics at the Framingham Offspring Study visit 6 (n = 2337)

Echocardiographic Measure	Adjusted for Age and BMI			Adjusted for Age Hypertension, BMI, Renal Dysfunction, Diabetes, Alcohol Use, Smoking, and Total Cholesterol to HDL Cholesterol Ratio		
	Gout	No Gout	P Value	Gout	No Gout	P Value
Mean LV thickness (cm)	2.02	1.89	<.0001	1.99	1.89	<.0001
Mean LV fractional shortening (range 0–1)	0.35	0.37	.006	0.35	0.37	.005
Mean LV diastolic internal dimension (cm)	5.00	4.79	<.0001	4.96	4.79	.003
Mean LV mass (g)	188.51	159.29	<.0001	182.47	159.58	<.001
Proportion of participants with systolic dysfunction (%)[a]	12.7	3.5	<.0001	10.0	2.3	.002
Proportion of participants with low ejection fraction (%)[a]	7.7	2.3	.001	5.3	1.6	.003

Hypertension was defined per the seventh report of the Joint National Committee on prevention, detection, evaluation, and treatment of high blood pressure (JNC 7) guidelines and/or use of anti-hypertensive medications. Diabetes was defined using the American Diabetes Association criteria or use of anti-diabetes medications.
  Abbreviations: HDL, high-density lipoprotein; LV, left ventricle.
  [a] Two-dimensional echocardiography was globally assessed by study physician for abnormal ejection fraction and evidence of mild or greater systolic dysfunction as assessed by visual assessment in multiple views.
  From Krishnan E. Gout and the risk for incident heart failure and systolic dysfunction. BMJ Open 2012;2(1):e000282.

Table 5
Mortality analyses by gout and heart failure status in the Framingham Offspring Study using Poisson regressions (n = 4989)

	Number of Observations in the Model	RR for Death (95% CI)
Unadjusted estimates		
Heart failure vs no heart failure	32,267	5.28 (4.89–5.69)
Gout vs no gout	32,267	1.74 (1.57–1.93)
Gout vs no gout among those without heart failure	30,774	1.55 (1.34–1.76)
Gout vs no gout among those with heart failure	1493	1.24 (1.02–1.51)
Adjusted estimates[a]		
Heart failure vs no heart failure	27,209	3.73 (3.39–4.10)
Gout vs no gout	27,209	1.58 (1.40–1.78)
Gout vs no gout among those without heart failure	26,073	1.50 (1.30–1.73)
Gout vs no gout among those with heart failure	1136	1.37 (1.10–1.74)

[a] Adjusted for age, BMI and total cholesterol to high-density lipoprotein ratio as continuous variables; and hypertension, BMI, renal dysfunction, diabetes, alcohol use, and smoking as categorical variables.

gout and increased cardiovascular risk. Farquharson and colleagues[31] assessed effect of allopurinol, the standard urate-lowering treatment of gout, in 11 normouricemic subjects (mean age, 67.5 years; 10 men, 1 woman) with CHF. They found that allopurinol improved endothelial function. The same group performed two randomized

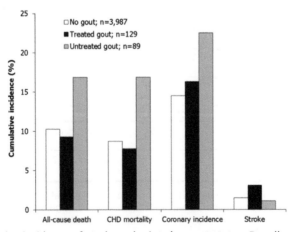

Fig. 6. Cumulative incidence of study endpoints by gout status. For all outcomes except stroke, the rates among gout subjects not on medication were significantly higher than for those without gout. Participants were considered treated for gout if they reported use of allopurinol, probenecid, or colchicine during the study. (*From* Krishnan E, Pandya BJ, Lingala B, et al. Hyperuricemia and untreated gout are poor prognostic markers among those with a recent acute myocardial infarction. Arthritis Res Ther 2012;14(1):R10.)

controlled trials to evaluate the effect of gout therapies on CHF.[32] They monitored endothelial function in 30 subjects (mean age, 69.7 years; 25 men, 5 women) with mild to moderate CHF treated with 300 mg allopurinol, 600 mg allopurinol, or placebo. Both dose levels of allopurinol improved endothelial function significantly better than placebo; the higher dose of allopurinol also improved endothelial function significantly better than the lower dose. The group then compared 1000 mg probenecid versus placebo in a study of 26 subjects with mild to moderate CHF (mean age, 67.0 years; 22 men, 4 women). Despite similar levels of urate lowering as observed with allopurinol, the uricosuric agent probenecid had no effect on endothelial function. Improvements in endothelial function thus seemed to be a result of a reduction in oxidative stress rather than the urate lowering.[32]

Noman and colleagues[33] in a double-blind, placebo-controlled, crossover trial assessed the antianginal effects of allopurinol in 65 subjects with stable angina pectoris and documented coronary artery disease. They found that xanthine oxidase inhibition by high-dose allopurinol (600 mg daily) improved objective measures of exercise-induced myocardial ischemia with a trend toward reducing anginal symptoms and sublingual glyceryl trinitrate use. Goicoechea and colleagues[34] studied the effect of allopurinol in chronic kidney disease progression and cardiovascular risk in a prospective, randomized trial of 113 subjects (57 in allopurinol group, 56 in control group) with renal disease. Over a mean follow-up time of 23.4 months, 22 subjects suffered a cardiovascular event: 15 in the control group and 7 in the allopurinol group. When adjusted for age, estimated glomerular filtration rate change, and serum uric acid levels, allopurinol treatment significantly decreased the risk of cardiovascular events (HR 0.29; 95% CI: 0.09–0.86). In another prospective, randomized clinical trial, Nidorf and colleagues[35] randomly assigned 532 subjects with stable coronary disease (on standard secondary prevention therapies) to colchicine (0.5 mg/d) and no colchicine groups. After a median of 3 years colchicine was shown to decrease significantly risk of cardiovascular events (HR = 0.33; 95% CI: 0.18–0.59).

POTENTIAL PATHOPHYSIOLOGIC PATHWAYS

There are several plausible mechanisms explaining the associations between gout and CVD (**Fig. 7**). The contribution of hyperuricemia to CVD risk has been postulated based on pathophysiologic mechanisms, including vascular smooth muscle cell proliferation and inflammation and platelet adhesiveness and aggregation. A recent meta-analysis found an independent impact of hyperuricemia on CHD risk; CHD risk increased by 9% in subjects with hyperuricemia.[36] Low-grade chronic inflammation associated with gout may also promote atherogenesis and thrombogenesis[37,38] based on other inflammatory arthritides that are also associated with increased risk of CVD.[39,40] The shared risk factors of male gender, age, diabetes, hypertension, obesity, alcohol consumption, metabolic syndrome, and menopause, which are common for both gout and CVD, constitute the indirect causal pathway for the association between gout and CVD. A recent study assessed the prevalence of cardiovascular risk factors among subjects attending a rheumatology outpatient clinic in comparison with the general population.[41] The investigators concluded that lifestyle-associated and potentially modifiable cardiovascular risk factors are overrepresented along the whole spectrum of chronic rheumatic diseases. Of these subjects, those with gout had higher prevalence of all cardiovascular risk factors studied, including current smoking (OR: 1.5; 95% CI: 1.0–2.3), hypertension (OR: 2.7; 95% CI: 1.7–4.3), abnormal cholesterol profile (OR: 1.5; 95% CI: 1.1–2.2), and obesity (OR: 4.7; 95% CI: 3.2–6.7).

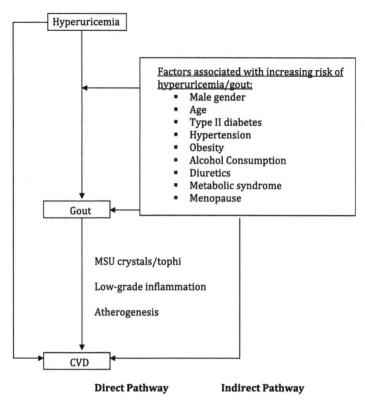

Fig. 7. Direct and indirect causal pathways linking hyperuricemia, gout, and CVD. MSU, monosodium urate.

The pathophysiologic pathways that link gout and myocardial dysfunction are unclear. The two major categories of heart failure are those caused by hypertension and those caused by atherosclerotic coronary artery disease. Gout is associated with both hypertension and CVD.[42] If the causality of association between gout and CVD are assessed, the association fulfills the following criteria of Bradford-Hill: (1) strength of association, (2) consistency across studies, (3) temporal sequence, (4) biologic rationale, and (5) coherence of findings. The limitations of the available data include lack of a clear-cut biologic gradient and lack of specificity of the gout-CVD link. Recent randomized controlled trials indicating that antigout medications lower the incidence of CVD provide experimental support for the causality theory. Furthermore, for multifactorial diseases such as CVD, specificity is not a criterion that needs to be fulfilled.

PUBLIC HEALTH SIGNIFICANCE AND SUMMARY

Over the last few decades, the burden of gout has increased substantially. The prevalence of self-reported, physician-diagnosed gout in the US adult population as estimated from the NHANES, 2007 to 2008, was 3.9% of the population (8.3 million individuals).[5] The prevalence among men was 5.9% (6.1 million) and that among women was 2.0% (2.2 million). These estimates were higher than those in NHANES III (1988–1994)[43] with differences of 1.2% in the prevalence of gout (95% CI: 0.6–1.9). The increasing burden of gout is observed worldwide.[44–50] A multicenter study of general practices in the United Kingdom reported that the prevalence of gout in 1991 had increased three-fold compared with the estimates from the 1970s.[46] Thus, even a small magnitude of risk elevation for CVD among these individuals can mean substantially higher absolute numbers of CVD in general population.

In addition to the burden due to elevated risk of CVD-related morbidity, significant mortality and costs in developed as well as developing countries result from gout. Gout is one of the most painful types of inflammatory arthritis, and patients are likely to seek immediate medical help when they suffer from a gout flare. In fact, gout is commonly diagnosed by primary care providers.[48] The diagnosis of gout should trigger the assessment of patient for cardiovascular risk factors and should lead to counseling and sensitization of patients about the future risk of CVD. The physician should specifically focus on the modifiable shared risk factors including diabetes, hypertension, obesity, metabolic syndrome, and intake of diuretics, because changes in these factors will help to control the severity of gout as well as prevent the morbidity and/or mortality owing to CVD. Finally, a significant body of clinical evidence indicates that aggressive management of gout using uricosuric drugs should be considered in individuals with high risk of CVD.

REFERENCES

1. Wu X, Muzny DM, Lee CC, et al. Two independent mutational events in the loss of urate oxidase during hominoid evolution. J Mol Evol 1992;34(1):78–84.
2. Ames BN, Cathcart R, Schwiers E, et al. Uric acid provides an antioxidant defense in humans against oxidant-and radical-caused aging and cancer: a hypothesis. Proc Natl Acad Sci U S A 1981;78(11):6858–62.
3. Krishnan E, Baker JF, Furst DE, et al. Gout and the risk of acute myocardial infarction. Arthritis Rheum 2006;54(8):2688–96.
4. Mateos Antón F, Garcia Puig J, Ramos T, et al. Sex differences in uric acid metabolism in adults: evidence for a lack of influence of estradiol-17 beta (E_2) on the renal handling of urate. Metabolism 1986;35(4):343–8.
5. Zhu Y, Pandya BJ, Choi HK. Prevalence of gout and hyperuricemia in the US general population: the National Health and Nutrition Examination Survey 2007–2008. Arthritis Rheum 2011;63(10):3136–41.
6. Bhole V, de Vera M, Rahman MM, et al. Epidemiology of gout in women: fifty-two–year followup of a prospective cohort. Arthritis Rheum 2010;62(4):1069–76.
7. Huchard H. Traite Clinique des Maladies du Coeur et de L'Aorta. 3rd edition. Paris: G. Doin; 1899.
8. Roberts W. Gout. In: Allbutt T, editor. A system of medicine by many writers. London: Macmillan; 1897. p. 160.
9. D'Agostino RB, Kannel WB. Epidemiological background and design: the Framingham Study. Proceedings of the American Statistical Association sesquicentennial invited paper sessions. 1989. p. 707–18.
10. Abbott RD, Brand FN, Kannel WB, et al. Gout and coronary heart disease: the Framingham Study. J Clin Epidemiol 1988;41(3):237–42.
11. Yü TA, Talbott JH. Changing trends of mortality in gout. Semin Arthritis Rheum 1980;10(1):1–9. Elsevier.
12. Nishioka K, Mikanagi K. A retrospective study on the cause of death, in Japan, of patients with gout. Ryumachi 1981;21:29.
13. Chen SY, Chen CL, Shen ML. Severity of gouty arthritis is associated with Q-wave myocardial infarction: a large-scale, cross-sectional study. Clin Rheumatol 2007;26(3):308–13.

14. Stamp LK, Wells JE, Pitama S, et al. Hyperuricaemia and gout in New Zealand rural and urban Māori and non-Māori communities. Intern Med J 2013;43(6): 678–84.
15. Winnard D, Wright C, Jackson G, et al. Gout, diabetes and cardiovascular disease in the Aotearoa New Zealand adult population: co-prevalence and implications for clinical practice. N Z Med J 2011;126(1368):53–64.
16. De Muckadell OB, Gyntelberg F. Occurrence of gout in Copenhagen males aged 40–59. Int J Epidemiol 1976;5(2):153–8.
17. Gelber AC, Klag MJ, Mead LA, et al. Gout and risk for subsequent coronary heart disease: the Meharry-Hopkins study. Arch Intern Med 1997;157(13):1436.
18. Krishnan E, Svendsen K, Neaton JD, et al. Long-term cardiovascular mortality among middle-aged men with gout. Arch Intern Med 2008;168(10):1104.
19. Choi HK, Curhan G. Independent impact of gout on mortality and risk for coronary heart disease. Circulation 2007;116(8):894–900.
20. De Vera MA, Rahman MM, Bhole V, et al. Independent impact of gout on the risk of acute myocardial infarction among elderly women: a population-based study. Ann Rheum Dis 2010;69(6):1162–4.
21. Teng GG, Ang LW, Saag KG, et al. Mortality due to coronary heart disease and kidney disease among middle-aged and elderly men and women with gout in the Singapore Chinese Health Study. Ann Rheum Dis 2012;71(6):924–8.
22. Kuo CF, See LC, Luo SF, et al. Gout: an independent risk factor for all-cause and cardiovascular mortality. Rheumatology 2010;49(1):141–6.
23. Kok VC, Horng JT, Lin HL, et al. Gout and subsequent increased risk of cardiovascular mortality in non-diabetics aged 50 and above: a population-based cohort study in Taiwan. BMC Cardiovasc Disord 2012;12(1):108.
24. Stack A, Hanley A, Casserly L, et al. Independent and conjoint associations of gout and hyperuricaemia with total and cardiovascular mortality. QJM 2013; 106(7):647–58.
25. Krishnan E. Hyperuricemia and incident heart failure. Circ Heart Fail 2009;2(6): 556–62.
26. Anker SD, Doehner W, Rauchhaus M, et al. Uric acid and survival in chronic heart failure validation and application in metabolic, functional, and hemodynamic staging. Circulation 2003;107(15):1991–7.
27. Zhu Y, Pandya BJ, Choi HK. Comorbidities of gout and hyperuricemia in the US General Population: NHANES 2007-2008. Am J Med 2012;125(7):679–87.e1.
28. Krishnan E. Gout and the risk for incident heart failure and systolic dysfunction. BMJ Open 2012;2(1):e000282.
29. Struthers A, Donnan P, Lindsay P, et al. Effect of allopurinol on mortality and hospitalisations in chronic heart failure: a retrospective cohort study. Heart 2002; 87(3):229–34.
30. Thanassoulis G, Brophy JM, Richard H, et al. Gout, allopurinol use, and heart failure outcomes. Arch Intern Med 2010;170(15):1358.
31. Farquharson CA, Butler R, Hill A, et al. Allopurinol improves endothelial dysfunction in chronic heart failure. Circulation 2002;106(2):221–6.
32. George J, Carr E, Davies J, et al. High-dose allopurinol improves endothelial function by profoundly reducing vascular oxidative stress and not by lowering uric acid. Circulation 2006;114(23):2508–16.
33. Noman A, Ang DS, Ogston S, et al. Effect of high-dose allopurinol on exercise in patients with chronic stable angina: a randomised, placebo controlled crossover trial. Lancet 2010;375(9732):2161–7.

34. Goicoechea M, de Vinuesa SG, Verdalles U, et al. Effect of allopurinol in chronic kidney disease progression and cardiovascular risk. Clin J Am Soc Nephrol 2010;5(8):1388–93.
35. Nidorf SM, Eikelboom JW, Budgeon CA, et al. Low-dose colchicine for secondary prevention of cardiovascular disease. J Am Coll Cardiol 2013;61(4):404–10.
36. Kim SY, Guevara JP, Kim KM, et al. Hyperuricemia and coronary heart disease: a systematic review and meta-analysis. Arthritis Care Res (Hoboken) 2010; 62(2):170–80.
37. Hansson GK. Inflammation, atherosclerosis, and coronary artery disease. N Engl J Med 2005;352(16):1685–95.
38. Epstein FH, Ross R. Atherosclerosis—an inflammatory disease. N Engl J Med 1999;340(2):115–26.
39. Solomon DH, Karlson EW, Rimm EB, et al. Cardiovascular morbidity and mortality in women diagnosed with rheumatoid arthritis. Circulation 2003;107(9): 1303–7.
40. Han C, Robinson DW, Hackett MV, et al. Cardiovascular disease and risk factors in patients with rheumatoid arthritis, psoriatic arthritis, and ankylosing spondylitis. J Rheumatol 2006;33(11):2167–72.
41. Meek IL, Picavet HSJ, Vonkeman HE, et al. Increased cardiovascular risk factors in different rheumatic diseases compared with the general population. Rheumatology 2013;52(1):210–6.
42. Krishnan E. Inflammation, oxidative stress and lipids: the risk triad for atherosclerosis in gout. Rheumatology 2010;49(7):1229–38.
43. Kramer HM, Curhan G. The association between gout and nephrolithiasis: the National Health and Nutrition Examination Survey III, 1988-1994. Am J kidney Dis 2002;40(1):37–42.
44. Arromdee E, Michet CJ, Crowson CS, et al. Epidemiology of gout: is the incidence rising? J Rheumatol 2002;29(11):2403–6.
45. Mikuls TR, Saag KG. New insights into gout epidemiology. Curr Opin Rheumatol 2006;18(2):199–203.
46. Harris CM, Lloyd DC, Lewis J. The prevalence and prophylaxis of gout in England. J Clin Epidemiol 1995;48(9):1153–8.
47. Klemp P, Stansfield SA, Castle B, et al. Gout is on the increase in New Zealand. Ann Rheum Dis 1997;56(1):22–6.
48. Kim KY, Ralph Schumacher H, Hunsche E, et al. A literature review of the epidemiology and treatment of acute gout. Clin Ther 2003;25(6):1593–617.
49. Zeng QY, Chen R, Darmawan J, et al. Rheumatic diseases in China. Arthritis Res Ther 2008;10(1):R17.
50. Chuang SY, Lee SC, Hsieh YT, et al. Trends in hyperuricemia and gout prevalence: nutrition and Health Survey in Taiwan from 1993-1996 to 2005-2008. Asia Pac J Clin Nutr 2011;20(2):301–8.
51. Darlington L, Slack J, Scott J. Vascular mortality in patients with gout and in their families. Ann Rheum Dis 1983;42(3):270–3.
52. Janssens H, Van de Lisdonk E, Bor H, et al. Gout, just a nasty event or a cardiovascular signal? A study from primary care. Fam Pract 2003;20(4):413–6.
53. Cohen SD, Kimmel PL, Neff R, et al. Association of incident gout and mortality in dialysis patients. J Am Soc Nephrol 2008;19(11):2204–10.
54. Kuo CF, Yu KH, See LC, et al. Risk of myocardial infarction among patients with gout: a nationwide population-based study. Rheumatology 2013;52(1):111–7.

Index

Note: Page numbers of article titles are in **boldface** type.

Rheum Dis Clin N Am 40 (2014) 145–154
http://dx.doi.org/10.1016/S0889-857X(13)00107-5
0889-857X/14/$ – see front matter © 2014 Elsevier Inc. All rights reserved.

rheumatic.theclinics.com

Printed and bound by CPI Group (UK) Ltd, Croydon, CR0 4YY

03/10/2024

01040488-0013